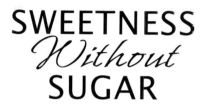

PRAISE FOR

SWEETNESS *Without* SUGAR

"*Sweetness Without Sugar* is a delightful resource for creating and enjoying healthy, delicious sweet-tasting foods. Wendy's book is a well-researched compilation of all she has learned, shared and believes in as a nutritionist, mother, healer and counselor. She provides supportive guidance in every nourishing word."

SUSAN TATE, M.A.
Author of *Wellness Wisdom: 31 Ways to Nourish Your
Mind, Body & Spirit* and *Into the Mouths of Babes*

"*Sweetness Without Sugar* is chock full of well-researched information and tasty recipes. My clients are always looking for the "how to" when making positive health changes. Hats off to Wendy for not compromising her message, but giving her readers the ability to make the necessary changes in a delicious way!"

**BONNIE C. MINSKY, MA, MPH, CNS, LDN,
NUTRITIONAL CONCEPTS INC.**
www.nutritionalconcepts.com

"*Sweetness Without Sugar* is a complete review of sugar, sugar-like products and products which are sweet but have none of the toxicity of sugar. It is an easy-to-read, practical guide for cooking with sugar replacements. The recipes are simple to make and taste delicious! In an age when we have come to realize that sugar is an enemy of health, Wendy Vigdor-Hess provides an easy guide for the masses. My dream is to have a copy of this book in each home economics class in our schools and on the shelves of good cooks everywhere. If our children ate these foods in place of traditional snacks and school lunches we would all grow up healthier!! Readers will discover how to reduce their risks of diabetes, heart disease and obesity after reading *Sweetness Without Sugar*. Thank you, Wendy, for a great guide!"

GREG GELBURD, M.D., FAMILY PRACTICE PHYSICIAN

"Ms. Vigdor-Hess has written an important and useful book. She offers practical and compelling advice to help readers decrease their sugar intake and improve their health. This book is a wonderful resource for anyone hoping to control their blood sugar, decrease inflammation and possibly even prevent serious diseases such as cancer."
DELIA CHIARAMONTE, M.D., PRESIDENT,
INSIGHT MEDICAL CONSULTANTS
www.insightmedicalconsultants.com

"For those wanting to stop eating sugar but still enjoy the healthy alternatives, this is an excellent guide book. For the recipes alone, this book is a "treat." The added features offer clear, comprehensive choices for sweetening alternatives for gluten-free, vegan baking."
LEIF GRUNSETH, ATC, CNMT, LMP, CERTIFIED ATHLETIC TRAINER,
Certified Neuromuscular Therapist, Licensed Massage Practitioner
www.leifgrunseth.com

"In *Sweetness Without Sugar*, Wendy offers a one-stop-shop for anyone dealing with negative effects from gluten, dairy, sugar or toxic sugar substitutes. More than just a cookbook, this resource guide empowers its readers to choose wisely without compromising taste. They'll learn the how's and why's of sugar sensitivity and healthy sweet treats. Smoothies, breakfasts, and both raw and baked desserts appeal to anyone watching a waistline or looking to raise vitality. In her warm, friendly way, Wendy nurtures as she educates. I've already referred many clients and friends to the eBook version and look forward to the print edition!"
LAURA BRUNO, LIFE COACH AND MEDICAL INTUITIVE
Author of *If I Only Had a Brain Injury, The Lazy Raw Foodist's Guide* and
Schizandra and the Gates of Mu
www.internationalrenaissancecoaching.com

"Wendy has created a useful and practical book that provides a wealth of information about sweeteners and organic alternatives. Her recipes for organic treats are a hit in our home. I recommend it as a good resource for anyone wishing to improve their health through balanced, natural nutrition."
MITCHELL A. FLEISHER, M.D., D.HT., D.A.B.F.M., Dc.A.B.C.T.
Author of *Alternative DrMCare Natural Medical Self-Care Protocols*
www.alternativedrmcare.com

"This book has been a gift to me both personally and professionally. I am using Wendy's recipes to feed my family more healthfully, and my patients are doing the same. So many of us battle with the allure of sugar in all of its forms. What a joy to be able to incorporate sweetness into our lives more nutritiously! I had tried many alternative sweetener recipes and was consistently disappointed with the results. Wendy's recipes are foolproof - each one I have tried is delicious (and my kids and patients agree!) This book is a must-read for anyone who is interested in a healthier lifestyle."
SANDI KAPLAN, MS, RD,
Assistant Director of Clinical Support for Free & Clear, Inc.
and Co-creator of Zingbars®
www.freeclear.com and *www.zingbars.com*

"I am thrilled to be able to recommend Wendy's book to my clients! So many people are looking for refined sugar alternatives, and Wendy has created such delicious, easy to prepare treats that everyone can enjoy. This book is more than a cookbook too…it is loaded with sound nutrition information. Thanks for putting this book out there! So many people will benefit from your wisdom and talents!"
KAREN RADEN, MS, RD, CCN, INTEGRATIVE NUTRITIONIST
www.karenraden.com

"Thank you for sending me your book, *Sweetness Without Sugar*. I do not recall reading another book on nutrition with the same enthusiasm. What a treasure trove of information! The book is a cornucopia of balanced, factual information on sugars, artificial sweeteners, corn, gluten, dairy, soy, essential fatty acids, etc. – even alkaline diet. What makes this book such a practical guide are the charts, tables, website references, and recipes, which fill almost two-thirds of the pages. I will recommend this book wholeheartedly to all my clients with a "sweet tooth". It will be a tremendous help for them to transition to a sugar-free diet without having to abstain from sweetness."
PETER HINDERBERGER, M.D., PH.D., INTEGRATIVE MEDICINE,
Anthroposophic Medicine, Homeopathy, Nutrition and Lifestyle

"What a wonderful group of fun recipes that are easy to make for the family! I love the variety of treats and that no one has to feel deprived while trying to optimize his or her children's health! Thank you for your contribution to our profession!"

KATHLEEN PUTNAM, MS, RD

Parent Coach and Owner of NutritionWorks Consulting

www.nutritionworkseattle.com

"As a holistic nutrition educator, I gear my learning and teaching toward whole natural foods that help create wellness. Wendy's new book, *Sweetness Without Sugar,* is a perfect fit for the families who come to see me. Her introduction to natural sugar substitutes with definitions will surely help wipe away the confusion about the many names used for sweeteners. She has such a wide blend of choices here from the raw foodist options, to vitality-rich smoothies, to more traditional baked goods like chocolate chip cookies. With such a range of choices, anyone could pick up this book and start at a level they are comfortable with, and expand their new ventures in creating sugar-free sweets at their own pace. What really pleases me is that Wendy uses healthy nutrient-dense nutritional boosters in many recipes, making them less of a splurge and more of a boost! Not to be overlooked is the introduction to each recipe, which describes how Wendy enjoys or uses each dish. The simple 'mom style' explanation of each recipe helps take something that may seem unfamiliar and gives it a useable space in daily food preparation. Well thought out, well-written, with something for everyone. I am glad to recommend *Sweetness Without Sugar* to my clients.

LAURA SCHMITT, NE

Certified Holistic Nutrition Educator specializing in allergies and whole foods

Published author, teacher, mother and Co-founder of

www.glutenanddairyfree.com

"This cookbook is the one I have been looking for to recommend to my families. So many cookbooks touted as "healthy" include soy products, margarine, corn products and high concentrates of natural sweeteners. Wendy's *Sweetness Without Sugar* provides friendly wisdom, the latest in nutritional and allergy facts, quick recipes that not only pass my taste and nutritional tests but the taste test of all four of my young children and the parents and toddlers in my practice. This is truly a whole food cook book which introduces natural and nutritious sweeteners that are slowly and easily absorbed and enjoyed. You will find child-friendly high-protein vegan treats in this book! After enjoying the recipes in this book, you and your family are sure to notice less allergies, chronic illnesses and behavioral issues. Be sure and keep this cookbook at your fingertips in the kitchen and plan to be inspired to properly stock (and purge) your cupboards."

DR. JENNIFER CURTIS PRAX, B.A., D.C., C.S.T., D.IC.C.P.
Board Certified Pediatric Chiropractor, Charlottesville, VA
International Chiropractic Association Council on Chiropractic Pediatrics
www.chiroprax.com

"This book is a concise, compact, easy-to-use encyclopedia and cookbook; a brilliant bridge from unhealthy sugar consumption. Individually, the various listings, categories and definitions are worth the purchase! Having raised six children on sugar-free diets, I understand the needs, temptations and social pressures of sugar in the marketplace. Because of the corn syrup revolution in the 1970's, Western culture has become not just addicted but scientifically proven to be neurologically hardwired and genetically predisposed to crave sugar. Even with global knowledge of the effects of sugar-laden diets and the epidemic of obesity, individuals have difficulty refraining from sugar consumption because they are tempted everywhere including health foods stores. *Sweetness Without Sugar* with its wonderful delicious-tasting, healthy alternative recipes, is a welcome addition to any home."

DARIA M. BREZINSKI, PH.D.
Educator, advocate, therapist, entrepreneur and author of
Reflecting Identity (poetry), *Defining Identity* (personal, community, global),
Molding Identity (educational system) and *Transcending Identity* (theology)
www.drdariabrezinski.com

Sweetness Without Sugar

2/11/2011: Red Planetary Moon (Purifies Universal Water Flow)

ISBN: 978-0-9845603-7-0

Printed in the United States by SolThea℠ Press

Edited by Traci Moore (*www.tracimoore.org*)

Book design by Gwen Gades (*www.beapurplepenguin.com*) and
Jasper Burns (*www.jasperburns.com*)

Cover design by Cathi Stevenson (*www.BookCoverExpress.com*)

Photography (viewed at *www.SweetnessWithoutSugar.com*) by
Sraddha VanDyke (*http://sraddha.weebly.com*)

Logo design by Jan Gulley Gerdin (*www.bring-design.com*)

Indexing by Clive Pyne (*www.cpynebookindexing.com*)

 If you are interested in attending one of my *Sweetness
Without Sugar* workshops, please contact me. I offer
nutritional consultations via phone and in-person to cater
to the individual needs of clients. My website addresses are
www.SweetnessWithoutSugar.com and *www.vigdorhess.com*.

Limits of Liability and Disclaimer of Warranty:

Printed on paper from sustainably managed forests.

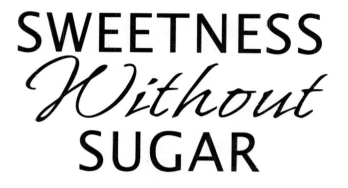

SWEETNESS *Without* SUGAR

A Resource Guide for Delicious
Dairy-, Egg- and Gluten-Free Treats
Made with Healthy Sweeteners

BY WENDY VIGDOR-HESS, RD

Dedication

I dedicate this book to people who want to choose a conscious
path and have the courage to live without relying on traditional
forms of sugar. I hope to inspire people to make more educated
decisions about the food they eat and in doing so, positively effect
manufacturing, food labeling and the quality of food produced.

May our children learn to find their inner sweetness, live
by it and allow it to shine forth...a prayer for us all.

*"There is a vitality, a life force, an energy, a quickening, that is translated
through you into action, and because there is only one of you in all time,
this expression is unique."*
– Martha Graham

SWEETNESS
Without
SUGAR

A Resource Guide for Delicious Dairy-, Egg- and Gluten-Free Treats Made with Healthy Sweeteners

BY WENDY VIGDOR-HESS, RD

Thank you for purchasing the second edition of *Sweetness Without Sugar*, a resource guide and cookbook for making delicious desserts from alternative sweeteners, dairy-, egg-, and gluten-free ingredients. This revised edition includes nutritional analyses for the recipes and additional chapters:

❋ Exploring the Reasons Behind the Reach
❋ Sweetness for Pre-Pregnancy, Pregnancy and Breastfeeding
❋ Corn, Corn Sugar and High Fructose Corn Syrup
❋ Sugar SAD: Sugar's Effects on Moods, Emotions and Weight

I've also included new website references, soaking and sprouting suggestions for nuts and seeds, recommended reading ideas and an informative chart to help you make wise choices about pesticides and conventional produce.

I'm presenting *Sweetness Without Sugar* in this form to offer you and your loved ones an economical resource for learning about sugar and for making sweet treats that are enjoyable to eat and good for your health.

Table of Contents

Author's Introduction

"Passion makes the old medicine new:
Passion lops off the bough of weariness.
Passion is the elixir that renews:
how can there be weariness
when passion is present?
Oh, don't sigh heavily from fatigue:
seek passion, seek passion, seek passion!"

\- Rumi

I'm delighted to share this resource guide with you. For as long as I can remember, I have loved sweets and chocolate. However, over the last seven years I recognized that my body and health do not love how I feel after eating sweets and chocolate. Consequently, I became passionate about finding ways to have sweetness in my life without the ill effects of eating traditional sugars.

Over time, many people have shared with me their addiction to sugar and their interest in reducing or eliminating their sugar dependency. People's insightful comments, questions and experiences have helped me expand my offerings to you. My *Sweetness Without Sugar* classes have also enhanced my education.

I learned that eating sugar hours or even days before nutritional coaching or Reiki sessions prevented me from offering the highest quality service possible. Although my intuition was still active, I felt "foggy" and, lethargic. Having a treat was no longer fun when my moods and "recovery" time were effected.

I want this guide to inspire you to make changes in your life. Many factors produce sweet cravings in people with and without known diseases like diabetes or hypoglycemia. This truth has fueled my curiosity and passion to provide resources for people who face this challenge.

Although sometimes described as a cookbook, *Sweetness Without Sugar* is written more as a resource guide for making gluten-free, vegan treats using alternative sweeteners. This book can function as a cookbook, as a guide for baking, and a resource for learning about food supply changes, for reading food labels and purchasing new products. The focus of this book is to explain the process of transitioning from processed sugars and artificial sweeteners to healthy natural sweeteners.

I have included many listings of products and websites to make it easier for you to find certain ingredients and save you time in researching purity and brand names. As of this printing, I feel confident with the recommendations regarding suppliers and products (see notations within sections). With our ever-changing economy and food policies, company owners and manufacturing processes may change. I encourage you to read the enclosed notations as well as investigate whether the foods meet your unique needs.

While investigating these topics, I noticed that most gluten-free and vegan baking books included common allergens (e.g. soy, corn) in addition to a lot of sugar. Most gluten-free baking also includes dairy products such as milk and eggs. Creating gluten-free and dairy-free recipes with alternative sweeteners has been a labor of love. I hope this book is valuable to you, your families and those you love.

It is in this vein that I also intend to inspire you to delve deep and find your unique sweetness. Taking the time to consider the positive experiences you enjoyed as a child can provide a portal to your heart's desires. Investigating your true passions and embracing what you truly love and can share in service to both yourself and the world, can alter your sugar cravings and bring you the sweetness you long for.

PART 1

Sweetness

Without Sugar

*Follow your bliss and the universe will open doors
where there were only walls.*

-Joseph Campbell

CHAPTER 1:

Sweetness

Without Sugar

Nothing but sweetness can remain when hearts are full of their own sweetness.
—William Butler Yeats

A Daily Dose

Many people would like to increase the amount of *sweetness* in their lives. With this book, rather than suggesting deprivation of sweets, I want to make it possible for you to enjoy your intake of healthy sweet treats in order to increase your inner *sweetness*.

The recipes included here offer sweet treats containing healthy nutrients. Incorporating a daily dose of these sweet items into your diet can reduce the likelihood of bingeing on unhealthy sweets or food, which can cause side effects, poor health and a negative self-image. My gluten-free, dairy-free and egg-free recipes also enhance your health and stimulate your healing journey. Recipes will appeal to people with a range of preferences including vegan, raw, allergen-free and even omnivorous diets.

This book is valuable for people who seek a continued guide towards optimal health, and for those who wish to adjust the form and quantity of their sweeteners. This book offers you healthy ways to bring *sweetness* into your life literally every day.

Finding Sweetness Within*

Unless you have chaos inside you, you cannot give birth to a dancing star.
— Nietzsche

How many times when reaching for those sweet treats have you paused to consider what effect you really want? Your choice of sugar may be repressing your true desire for happiness or joy, your innate *sweetness*. Some people use eating as a "drug" to deal with the lack of *sweetness* in their lives. Sugars contribute to this effect by causing low serotonin levels in the brain, which in turn lead to cravings for sweets and carbohydrates.

The average American consumes his weight in sugar every year (152 lbs). Sugar consumption has been linked directly to obesity, the most urgent health challenge to nutritional health during the 21st century. Research has also linked sugar intake to higher risks for diabetes, tooth decay, mood swings, lowered immunity and the loss of vital minerals from the body.

The form of sugar you choose can have a direct effect on your brain chemistry and blood sugar. Simple sugars (e.g. candy, corn syrup, refined flours, and starches) are highly glycemic, meaning they break down and enter the bloodstream immediately and cause blood sugar to ebb and flow more violently. These sugars often leave the blood sugar level lower than it was before eating. Consequently, your body falsely thinks it is out of fuel, resulting in hunger and a craving for more carbohydrates.

Sugar and corn syrup found in soft drinks, fruit drinks and sports drinks now supply more than ten percent of our total daily calories. Overloading on highly sweetened foods such as sports bars, candy and cookies also contributes to this cycle. These foods offer empty calories (e.g. no nutritional value), unhealthy fillers, chemicals, sugar and/or artificial sweeteners and they set us up for the next craving. Artificial sweeteners that are derived from chemicals — such as aspartame (Nutrasweet® or Equal®), sucralose (Splenda®), and saccharin — remain controversial given their possible long-term health consequences. While many people consume artificial sweeteners to limit their consumption of calories from traditional sugars, this practice may actually cause an increase in the consumption of sweets.

---

*   *A version of this article written by Wendy Vigdor-Hess was published in May of 2005, in* The Daily Progress *"Vital Signs Health Column", Charlottesville, Virginia.*

A study cited in the *International Journal of Obesity* revealed that eating artificially-sweetened foods and drinking sweetened beverages could hinder the body's ability to estimate caloric intake, thus boosting the inclination to overindulge on both artificially-sweetened foods *and* products sweetened with sugar. Eating large amounts of both sugar and artificial sweeteners suppresses the appetite for nourishing foods. This can cause not only weight gain and obesity, but also nutritional deficiencies. The human body is meant to consume more complex carbohydrates found in whole fruit, green vegetables, whole grains, and beans. Due to their fiber, vitamin and mineral content, these foods take time for the body to break down into simple sugars. To read the full article, visit: http://www.nature.com/ijo/journal/v28/n2/full/0802560a.html.

Some alternative sweeteners that our bodies recognize as complex carbohydrates are healthier for us than refined sugar. As with all sweeteners, these alternate forms are best eaten in moderation. They include fruit, coconut sugar, date sugar, 100% fruit concentrate, Rapadura® and stevia. Other natural alternative sweeteners like yacon, honey and maple syrup are derived directly from natural sources, and they act more like simple sugars in our bodies. As such, they are solid alternatives to refined sugar and processed sweeteners, although they should be consumed in moderation according to my recommendations on pages 92-93.

You can find alternative sweeteners in the baking or health food section of many local grocery or health food stores. If you don't find the ingredients, flours or sweeteners listed in the recipes, inquire about placing a special order at your local store.

To order superfoods or supplemental ingredients which may not be available locally, please see the websites noted in the *Appendix and Resources* section, or contact me.

Another way to reduce the amount of unwanted sweeteners in your diet is by reading food labels. If sugar or another sweetener, such as corn syrup, high fructose corn syrup, fructose (levulose), sucrose or dextrose are among the first few ingredients listed, look for another product that is less sweet.

Reaching for sugar may hinder your ability to take responsibility for what you want in life. The reasons behind the reach are as important as the reach for sugar itself. Acknowledging the truth about your cravings can do wonders for any waistline. Living our lives as kind, compassionate beings whose blood flows with innate *sweetness* is a gift to everyone— to ourselves, our loved ones and our communities.

> *Something we were withholding made us weak*
> *Until we found it was ourselves.*
>
> - Robert Frost

CHAPTER 2:

Sweets

And Health Implications

When you come looking for sugar,
Your bag will be examined
To see how much it can hold;
It will be filled accordingly.

-Rumi

n 1689, when the first sugar refinery was built, people consumed four pounds of sugar per year. The average amount of sugar that an American consumes per year equates to a half- pound, or roughly one cup, per day. One suggested goal is to consume less than ten pounds of sugar per year. The American Heart Association recently released its recommendations for our daily sugar intake: 140 kilocalories (about 35 grams) for most American men and 100 kilocalories (about 25 grams) for most American women (depending on age and activity level). These were considered the "prudent upper limits."

It is a well-known fact that sugar is added to baked goods, sweets and soda (ten teaspoons per ten-ounce can). However, manufacturers now add sugar to a wide variety of foods including lunch meats, packaged and prepared foods, low-fat foods and more. Food labeling mandates that the ingredients of highest concentration are listed first. If more sugar is contained in the product than any other, it must be listed first on the label.

One item not found on a food label that effects our bodies' response to sugar is glycemic index (GI). Glycemic index measures how carbohydrate foods affect blood glucose levels. Easily-digested carbohydrates like white bread and potatoes that release glucose rapidly into the bloodstream have a high glycemic index. In comparison, most vegetables, when digested, release glucose slowly into the bloodstream, and they consequently have a low GI. Choosing foods with a glycemic index value below 75 is ideal for most people who want to regulate their sugar cravings. However, those who struggle with more complex blood sugar issues may require more specialized guidance than glycemic index. Investigating your personal metabolic type, sensitivity to fructose and level of alkaline balance are other important steps. For more information about alkaline balance see pages 33-34.

Manufacturers have discovered that by including a variety of sweeteners in their products they can disguise the fact that a large portion of the product is made from sugar. As a result, consumers need to educate themselves about the different names for sugar. For more information see my list on pages 12-13.

When in a hurry or shopping with kids, many are duped into thinking the products they buy are healthy. For example, many yogurts sold today (even those sold in health food stores) often contain a variety of sweeteners. Even if you don't think you like or eat many sweets, you are likely exposed to many sugars daily.

Sweets and sugar have long been implicated in certain disease states such as frequent colds and flu, diabetes, hypo- or hyperglycemia and cavities. The Centers for Disease Control and Prevention estimate that one third of all American children who were born in the year 2000 will develop diabetes as a result of poor diet and lack of exercise. For the first time, statistics indicate that children may have a shorter life expectancy than their parents. One in four Americans has diabetes. Our nation spends $174 billion dollars per year on diabetes, which is about equal to the combined amount spent to date on the wars in Iraq, Afghanistan and the global war on terror.

The rising trend in obesity suggests that Americans are currently at their heaviest weight in history. Figures show that obesity (66% of the population) costs the American economy $75 billion per year. One out of three children and one of four teenagers are overweight or at risk. In 2006, the Centers for Disease Control reported that obesity kills more than 112,000 American citizens a year.

As of 2001, the National Soft Drink Association (NSDA) reported that the average American consumes over 600 12-ounce servings of soda per year! These figures point to a direct relationship between sugar consumption and childhood obesity, caffeine and sugar addiction, calcium loss from phosphoric acid (associated with bone loss), nutritional deficiencies, blood sugar disorders and tooth decay.

Marketing can play a large role in our children's choices. Research has shown that the risk for obesity increases 6% for every hour of television a pre-schooler watches per day. And considering that children view on average 51 hours of food ads every year (95% of them for "junk food"), one may choose to limit television time especially during cartoon programs when the same advertisement for a sugary food is broadcast every five minutes. Though making these changes may not be easy, the changes will have a positive long-term impact.

More recently, further correlations between sugar, artificial sweeteners and a multitude of health conditions have been exposed. Examples of *some* of these conditions include:

- Acid reflux or GERD
- ADD/ADHD
- Addictions
- Balance issues
- Cancer
- Candida yeast syndrome
- Cardiovascular disease
- Childhood obesity
- Colds and flu
- Cravings for more sugar and sweets!!
- Dehydration
- Depression
- Dizziness
- Fructose malabsorption and/or disorder
- GI disorders
- Headaches — including migraines
- Heart infections
- High blood pressure (Hypertension)
- High cholesterol
- Infertility
- Insomnia and other sleep disturbances
- Irritable bowel syndrome
- Kidney stones
- Low protein
- Memory loss
- Mental confusion (or "brain fog")
- Metabolic syndrome
- Mood swings
- Neurological damage and/or neurotoxins
- Obesity
- Osteoporosis
- Periodontitis — inflammation of the gums
- Poor digestion
- Poor mineral absorption
- Sexual dysfunction
- Skin eruptions or irritations
- Weight fluctuations

A study in the *Journal of the American Dietetic Association* (August 2009, Volume 109, Number 8) found a possible correlation between increased body weight and prolonged insulin resistance in cancer survivors. The results of this study stress the importance of balancing insulin. This balance could be applied to a variety of "populations" such as people who are obese or living with cancer. This research also demonstrates potential for disease prevention and positive outcomes when insulin levels are balanced.

In a recent study in *Nutrition and Metabolism* (April 9, 2010), Professors Thomas Seyfried and Laura Shelton hypothesize that "cancer is primarily a disease of energy metabolism." They demonstrate a connection between glucose and tumor growth, and that reducing calories and consumption of foods with more available glucose (e.g. high glycemic carbohydrates and sugar) also reduces levels of certain hormones active during cancer growth, thereby slowing the growth of cancer. Findings indicated that incorporating lean protein and healthy fats (e.g. omega 3 fatty acids) into the diet (instead of obtaining it from more glucose) will foster healthier growth of normal cells. I advise working with a health professional to assess personal dietary needs, and to ensure that one's daily caloric intake is balanced and nutrient-dense.

A well-known cross sectional study, the *National Health and Nutrition Examination Survey* (NHANES), has investigated the health factors of more than 6000 American adults over a seven-year period. The study associated markers of metabolic syndrome (such as low HDL and elevated triglycerides) with consumption of at least one soft drink per day. The analysis also indicated that a statistically significant health risk was associated with higher sugar consumption (e.g. from carbohydrates including soft drinks). These findings were applicable for soft drinks containing either sugar or artificial sweeteners.

As noted on the previous page, sugar has been shown to contribute to a variety of health conditions. Candida albicans or candida yeast syndrome is one such condition defined as a yeast infestation or fungus from a parasite that thrives in warm environments. It grows mostly in the intestines and can also be found in other organs. Addressing candida (and common problems associated with it) has helped reverse troublesome symptoms in numerous conditions, including autism, ADD/ADHD, fibromyalgia, and thyroid diseases.

Innately, we crave sweets. Sometimes cravings are the body's way of seeking balance. Craving sweets may also be a signal that the body needs hydration or protein. Consuming regular amounts of filtered water can help offset cravings and provide help for many common symptoms such as headaches, fatigue and mental "fogginess". If you are reading this and are a vegan or vegetarian, it is important to provide your body with adequate amounts of protein to both curtail sweet cravings and also to optimize your health.

Just as our brain may mistakenly believe sugar fulfills our craving for sweet, our body likely knows better. One example among menstruating women is that "monthly chocolate craving." Magnesium levels drop prior to menstruation, and chocolate is high in magnesium.

As babies, the first taste we experience is sweet, whether from breast milk or formula. "Sweet" is one of the five taste sensations (sweet, salty, sour, bitter and savory). Sweetness is here to stay in our lives and shifting toward more healthy alternatives is a positive and attainable goal. We can meet this goal and find more balance by replacing manufactured and processed sweeteners with more wholesome choices.

Reasons We Find It Difficult to Omit Sugar from Our Diets:

The Many Names for Sugar and Sweeteners

Many of these sweeteners are described in detail on pages 74-90.

- Agave (or agave nectar)
- Barbados sugar
- Barley malt
- Beet sugar
- Brown rice syrup
- Brown sugar
- Buttered syrup
- Cane juice crystals
- Cane sugar
- Caramel
- Carob syrup
- Castor sugar
- Corn sugar
- Corn syrup
- Corn syrup solids
- Crystalline dextrose
- Crystalline fructose
- Date sugar
- Dehydrated sugar cane juice (or dried)
- Demerara (common in the United Kingdom)
- Dextran
- Dextrose (same as monohydrate or anhydrous dextrose)
- Diastatic malt
- Diatase
- Disaccharides
- Dried cane juice
- Erythritol (corn-derived)
- Ethyl maltol
- Evaporated cane juice
- Florida Crystals®
- Fructose (found in fruit and sold in granulated form)
- Fruit juice
- Fruit juice concentrate
- Fruitsource®
- Galactose
- Glucose
- Glucose solids
- Glucose syrup
- Golden sugar
- Golden syrup
- Grape sugar
- High fructose corn syrup (HFCS)
- Honey
- Hydrogenated starch hydrolysates (HSH) derived from corn, wheat or potato
- Hydrolysed starch
- Invert sugar
- Invert syrup
- Isomalt
- Just Like Sugar®
- Lactitol
- Lactose
- Lakanto™
- Levulose
- Malt
- Maltitol
- Maltisorb™
- Maltisweet™ *
- Maltodextrin
- Maltol
- Maltose
- Malt syrup
- Mannitol
- Maple syrup
- Molasses
- Monosaccharides
- Muscovado sugar
- Mushroom sugar
- Mycose
- Organic Zero™
- Panocha
- Polydextrose
- Polysaccharides

(continued on next page)

*See page 82 for other sweeteners containing corn like Maltisweet™.

- Powdered sugar (also called confectioner's sugar)
- PureVia™
- Raffinose
- Rapadura®
- Raw sugar
- Refiners syrup
- Rice syrup
- Sorbitol
- Sorghum
- Sorghum syrup
- Stevia in the Raw™
- Sucanat®
- Sucrose
- Sugar
- Sugaridextrose
- Sugar in the Raw®
- Sun Crystals®
- Sweet Simplicity®
- Thaumatin
- TheraSweet™
- Treacle
- Trehalose
- The Ultimate Sweetener®
- Truvia™
- Turbinado sugar (more prevalent in United States)
- Xylitol
- Yellow sugar
- Z Sweet®

The Many Names for Artificial Sweeteners

- Acesulfame potassium
- Acesulfame K
- Ace-K
- Aclame™
- Alitame
- Altern™
- AminoSweet®
- Aspartame (aspartic acid plus phenylalanine plus methanol)
- Aspartic Acid
- Canderel®
- Cyclamate
- DiabetiSweet®
- Equal®
- Naturlose™
- Neohesperidin dihydrochalcone or NHDC
- Neotame™
- Novasweet™
- Nutrasweet®
- Nutrasweet 2000®
- P-4000
- Phenylalanine
- Saccharin
- Shugr™
- Splenda®
- Spoonful®
- Sucralose
- SugarTwin®
- Sunett®
- Sweet & Safe®
- Sweetener 2000®
- Sweet N' Low®
- Sweet One®
- Swiss Sweet®
- Tagatose
- Talin™

Following is a list of brand names and the artificial sweeteners their products contain:

❋ Aclame™ contains alitame.

❋ Altern™ contains sucralose and is a Wal-Mart Stores Inc. store-brand version of Splenda®.

- ❈ AminoSweet® contains aspartame (aspartic acid plus phenylalanine).

- ❈ Canderel® contains aspartame (aspartic acid plus phenylalanine).

- ❈ DiabetiSweet® contains isomalt (a sugar alcohol) and acesulfame potassium.

- ❈ Equal® contains aspartame (aspartic acid plus phenylalanine).

- ❈ Naturlose™ contains tagatose.

- ❈ Neotame™ contains aspartic acid and phenylalanine and is made by Nutrasweet®. It is known as E961 in Europe.

- ❈ Novasweet™ contains alitame.

- ❈ Nutrasweet® contains aspartame (aspartic acid plus phenylalanine).

- ❈ Nutrasweet 2000® contains aspartame (aspartic acid plus phenylalanine).

- ❈ P-4000 refers to a class of synthetic (chemical) sweeteners.

- ❈ Shugr™ includes erythritol, maltodextrin, tagatose and sucralose.

- ❈ Splenda® contains sucralose (which is a sugar molecule with chlorine added to it).

- ❈ Spoonful® contains aspartame (aspartic acid plus phenylalanine).

- ❈ SugarTwin® contains saccharin.

- ❈ Sunett® contains acesulfame-K.

- ❈ Sweet & Safe® contains acesulfame-K (sometimes noted as Sweet-N-Safe®).

- ❈ Sweetener 2000® contains aspartame (aspartic acid plus phenylalanine).

- ❈ Sweet N' Low® contains saccharin and cyclamate.

- ❈ Sweet One® contains acesulfame-K.

- ❈ Swiss Sweet® contains acesulfame-K.

- ❈ Talin™ contains thaumatin.

These sweeteners are found in many products such as chewing gum, sodas, beverages, fruit juices, jams and jellies, ice creams, frozen desserts, baking mixes, processed and/or canned fruits, puddings, pie fillings, salad dressings, sandwich

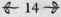

spreads, processed coffees and teas, dairy products and many baked goods!

Many processed and artificial sweeteners are supported by "big business." Large companies such as G.D. Searle & Company, Johnson & Johnson Services, The Monsanto Company, DuPont, Abbott Laboratories, The Coca-Cola Company, PepsiCo, and Cargill have been involved in some way with the "sweetener industry." The majority of artificial sweeteners on the list (on page 13) have been approved by the FDA in part because of the financial backing and reputations of these companies.

Though the focus of this book is to provide ways to enjoy sweets without the detrimental effects of processed sugars and artificial sweeteners, I'd like to offer a few key reasons why artificial sweeteners aren't healthy alternatives to sugar. Like sugar, corn syrup and soy, artificial sweeteners have been added to many common items in our food supply. They are man-made chemical creations, void of vitamins and minerals, and aren't truly safe for human consumption.

A category of artificial additives called excitotoxins are not beneficial to humans. Excitotoxins have been shown to destroy certain types of brain cells. Examples of excitotoxins are aspartame (an artificial sweetener found in NutraSweet® and Equal®), MSG, and hydrolyzed vegetable protein.

Excitotoxins have been shown to stimulate appetite and cravings. In an attempt to "meet the needs of their consumers", manufacturers have added excitotoxins to processed foods to make products taste "better." These toxins are often listed on product labels as general ingredients such as "spices, textured protein, natural flavoring", etc. Though some sensitive individuals may experience immediate symptoms, excitotoxins usually create disorders and brain damage over time. Liquid excitotoxins, found in sauces, gravies and other liquids are absorbed more rapidly.

For your convenience, here is a list of common ingredients (as noted on food labels) that may signify excitotoxins:

❀ Aspartame (NutraSweet® and Equal® and see lists on pages 13-14)

❀ Aspartate

❀ Aspartic acid

❀ Calcium caseinate

❀ Caseinate

❀ Cysteic acid

List of common ingredients that may signify excitotoxins (continued):

- ❈ Glutamate
- ❈ Glutamic acid
- ❈ Hydrolyzed plant protein
- ❈ Hydrolyzed vegetable protein
- ❈ MSG
- ❈ Natural flavoring
- ❈ Sodium caseinate
- ❈ Soy protein extract
- ❈ Spices
- ❈ Textured protein
- ❈ Vegetable protein
- ❈ Yeast extract

If you would like to learn more about this subject, I suggest reading *Excitotoxins: The Taste That Kills* by Russell L. Blaylock, MD, and *Sweet Deception* by Dr. Joseph Mercola. Additional DVD suggestions are noted in the *Appendix and Resources* section on page 315.

CHAPTER 3:

Exploring

the Reasons Behind the Reach

*The blessings for which we hunger are not to
be found in other places or people.*

*These gifts can only be given to you by yourself.
They are at home in the hearth of your soul.*

-John O'Donohue

As noted in Chapter 1, the reasons behind the reach are as important as the reach for sugar itself. The fact that sugar is so readily available in a variety of forms does not make our sugar journey any easier. The opiate and other physiological effects associated with insulin, leptin and bodily functions also make it challenging for humans to quench their desire for sweetness. In addition to these physiological realities, one's addictive reach for sugar may reflect unrealized inner desires.

After reading the first edition of *Sweetness Without Sugar*, a reader shared what she loved about the book. In addition to the charts, scientific information and recipes, she enjoyed understanding that the whole book focused on *sweetness* and how we find it on our own. It took me more than seven years to complete my journey towards sweetness, and this reader's astute perception summarized a key component of my experience.

When beginning my *sweetness* journey, I had no idea it would become a book. But after sharing my experiences, I happily witnessed others transform as they discovered their hidden sweetness. Being present for their "light bulb moments" – excited exclamations, tears of joy, times of letting go, and movement forward – has been extremely rewarding.

My passion for helping others see their unique beauty has been an important thread in re-weaving their relationship with sugar. In this book, I invite you to investigate areas in your life (that may be clouded by sugar haze) where you may wish to take more responsibility. By acknowledging your cravings (while addressing the physical and physiological realities of these cravings), you can uncover exciting truths about yourself. This investigation can begin at any age.

I commonly advise parents and soon-to-be-parents to discuss their thoughts with me about eating, sugar, treats, and offering food as a reward or punishment. Even conscious parenting delves into areas that can result in frustration, reluctance and other emotions. Though honest communication is not always comfortable, a lot of pertinent information can be gleaned if we recognize knowledge as a powerful tool.

Addressing situations without judgment of ourselves or others, and embracing discomfort surrounding those questions can be freeing and beneficial. I've found that these discussions tend to illuminate subjects people are curious about but might not address on their own. With the added incentive of becoming better role models for their children, parents often demonstrate courage, strength and determination.

Any observations and lessons learned act as beacons of light. Openly expressing what you desire for your children (however different from your current situation) will create positive movement forward. Although taking steps to change habits may feel like "moving in the dark", having the desire to change can motivate you to create new pathways toward health for you and your family.

After having many beneficial discussions with clients, I've learned that it can still be difficult for us to imagine the rewards for taking responsibility for our sugar cravings. Information about the rewards may not be appealing enough to us to change our ways. For example, even if we are told that changing our diets will result in great clarity - illuminating what we truly want or need in place of sugar - this may not be enough of an incentive for some of us to make the switch. A more "magical" incentive can come from taking small steps toward change, noticing our personal growth, and gradually seeing troublesome symptoms disappear. Finding what motivates us personally is enormously helpful. Also, sharing this journey with a friend, family member or loved one will make the change easier. The saying "It's the journey, not the destination" suggests that possibilities lie within when we embrace our personal journey, and, ultimately, ourselves.

We are fortunate to live during a time in history when many people want to improve the environment, the planet and themselves. Although change can sometimes be a challenge, it can also bring forth many new and fruitful (a.k.a. *sweet*) beginnings.

To help you explore your personal reasons behind your reach for sugar, consider the questions below. I advise addressing the questions on paper when you feel relaxed and calm. You may find it helpful to return to these questions at different stages in your *sweetness* journey. Also, having your answers on paper will allow you to measure your progress after you make life changes.

1. Do you notice certain situations when you often reach for sugar more than others (e.g. social situations or when feeling vulnerable, lonely, insecure, unhappy, angry, or bored)? For example, what is your "routine" around eating sweets at home? Do you come home after a long day and eat sweets in front of the television? Perhaps you eat sweets when you "wind down" in your pj's, when you catch up with a friend on the phone? Or at work, do you pass a bowl of candy, and, without thinking about it, grab a piece or handful? Explain.

2. What items do you reach for (e.g. chocolate, donuts, baked goods, lollipops, gummy-type candy, bread, etc.)? Is there a reason why you choose these items over others? Explain.

3. What memories do you recall about your childhood relationship with sweets (e.g. you weren't allowed sweets, they were always around, or they were given as a reward, etc.)? For instance, do you or did you often bake with family members? Did you have a cookie or candy jar at home? Do you talk with family members now about food, sweets, or recipe ideas? Was going out to the candy store a special occasion or a part of your regular routine? When you did well in a sport or on a test, were you taken out for a treat? Explain.

4. Do you enjoy eating what you choose? Do you taste it while eating it or eat it so quickly you don't even notice? Explain.

5. Are you aware of something you may need instead of the sugary item (e.g. extra sleep, a hug, attention, recognition, time to yourself, a break, a boost in energy, etc.)? Explain.

6. Are there things that you've always wanted to do that you are unable to give yourself? Consider creating a list of things that have blocked the way (e.g. responsibilities, money, health, family obligations, etc.). If the roadblocks on your list were removed, what would you do? (For example, if your bills and debt were paid, your health was great, you had no fear and you had a strong supportive system urging you to do and be what you wanted, what would you do?) Explain.

7. If you could share a particular quality about yourself that you're proud of, what would it be? Have you ever shared these qualities with others? If not, how often would you feel comfortable displaying these facets of your true essence? Often times some of our unique qualities are hidden behind others' expectations. Giving ourselves permission to share is a huge step towards embracing our sparkly, quirky, and special qualities. Explain.

8. What are some ways you enjoy taking care of yourself (e.g. walking in nature, exercising, talking with a friend, taking a bath, reading, creative outlets, etc.)? Take a few minutes (or more) to brainstorm about what brings you joy and relaxation. If there has been a time in your life where you felt flow, what helped create that? What details about this time felt significant to you? Did you do anything differently? What kinds of activities help you slow down and feel good? For instance, does it make you feel good to remember to take your vitamins or put on a meaningful necklace, organize a list, prepare early for the next day, or write in a journal? All of these things may seem "silly", but they may be very important to your state of well-being and your motivation for being productive in other areas of your life. Explain.

There are many reasons why we may not claim what we want in life. It is common to find that we weren't conscious about our choices. There are no right answers, just personal ones. Letting go of the "what ifs" (if = I fail) and replacing them with "what is" (is = I succeed) can be a powerful and wondrous experience.

I hope this book will serve as a stepping stone for embracing every part of your journey toward wellness, healing and vibrant health.

CHAPTER 4:

Sweetness

for Pre-Pregnancy, Pregnancy and Breastfeeding

Wisdom begins in wonder.

-Socrates

I often hear from parents who are frustrated with their child's love of candy, soda and anything sweet. Humans are predisposed to enjoy a sweet taste, so it is no surprise to hear that children also do. A common reality is the similarity between the parents' and the child's sweet food cravings.

Though a majority of family-planning books often discuss the importance of maintaining a healthy diet throughout a woman's pregnancy, they omit guidelines for removing artificial sweeteners and unhealthy sweets from the mother's diet. Most pregnancy books also fail to address dietary habits both parents should consider when preparing to raise children.

When a couple discusses their desire for starting a family, they may feel joy, anticipation and excitement. *Sweetness* is a necessary ingredient when preparing for pregnancy. A varied diet with healthy quantities of protein, fat, and carbohydrates is as important for the soon-to-be-mom as for the growing baby.

On the following pages are some suggestions you may want to consider when planning to have a child.

PRE-PREGNANCY

❋ Four to six months prior to "trying to get pregnant," remove artificial sweeteners and refined white sugar from your diet. Unfortunately, these sweeteners are found in many commonly recommended pregnancy foods such as yogurt, nausea-regulating candies, soda and starchy foods.

❋ Ask your doctor or midwife for a CBC to test your fasting blood glucose. The ideal range is between 70-80.

❋ If you haven't already done so, gather more information about your food sensitivities prior to conceiving. Research ways to minimize your food allergies. These steps will help you make wise food choices during pregnancy, the postpartum period and when preparing food for your little ones. Individual counseling is advised.

❋ Please see the tips on pages 56-57 to help you determine if eating nuts during these unique stages is appropriate for you.

❋ An optional but perhaps helpful test is the C-Reactive Protein (CRP). This test measures the amount of inflammation in your system. Higher inflammation may indicate food sensitivities and may affect fertility.

❋ Check your acid/alkaline balance with pH test strips (bought at your local health food store). This is recommended for both partners. Too much acid can kill sperm. Just as an alkaline environment decreases sweet cravings for you, it is also a wonderful environment for your growing baby.

❋ If you eat soy, choose fermented versions of tempeh or miso. If you eat tofu, choose only organic, non-GMO tofu (1x per week). Avoid all other soy items, especially if having infertility challenges. If you feel more comfortable avoiding all soy during this time period, do so, but also check food labels for hidden soy ingredients. Discuss this with your partner and health care practitioners to determine if soy is "right" for you at this special time: (*See* Chapter 9 *on pages 49-54 for more information on soy.*)

❊ Incorporate more healthy omega oils into your diet. (*See Chapter 7 on pages 35-40 for more information.*) These oils are healthy for you and great for reducing inflammation, balancing blood sugar and for your growing baby's brain development.

❊ Other conditions that may effect fertility are celiac disease and wheat/gluten sensitivity. There are blood tests used to determine if you or your partner have celiac disease. In addition, "gene tests" can also be used to exclude celiac disease, especially if blood results are somewhat inconclusive. If you are concerned about or experiencing infertility, consider avoiding gluten and/or having a test to rule out celiac disease. (*To learn more about wheat and/or gluten sensitivities, please see* Chapter 10 *on pages 55-66.*)

❊ Though the recipes in this book are dairy-free, if you eat dairy, switch to organic dairy sources to minimize consumption of allergens, hormones and antibiotics given to cattle.

PREGNANCY:

❊ If someone in your family has a severe food allergy (e.g. anaphylaxis reaction) or has been diagnosed with celiac disease, avoid or greatly minimize your intake of that particular food while pregnant and breastfeeding. If you are a mother-to-be who has a severe food allergy, you should definitely avoid the foods that cause severe reactions. (*To learn more about food allergies and sensitivities, please see* Chapter 10 *on pages 55-66.*)

❊ Women with morning sickness should choose snacks containing complex carbohydrates with a balance of healthy fat and/or protein. Avoid refined carbohydrates such as pastries, sweets, processed crackers and pretzels, which are often recommended in many pregnancy books. Replace these with whole grain foods such as brown rice or millet (and crackers or pretzels with those ingredients). Though these starchy foods may be comforting during this stage, I recommend incorporating nutrient-dense snack foods along with these "comforts." Some examples include hummus or bean spread with whole grain crackers, or brown rice with greens and beans.

❋ Prepare healthy grab-and-go snacks that taste good to you (such as the *Nut Balls* on page 136 or *Quinoa Fruit Muffins* on page 210). When tired and craving sugar, you will have these snacks available. If necessary, ask friends and family to help you prepare treats that you can freeze or have on hand when you are hungry.

❋ Choose only from your list of "tolerated" foods that you know will allow you to feel good after eating. If you find that you crave things other than your "usual" staples, choose the most wholesome food that you can tolerate and let the judgment go. *During my first pregnancy, when I told my husband I couldn't eat the vegetables I normally adored, my husband gave me a loving look and said, "Who are you?"*

❋ Sugar and sweet foods can contribute to morning sickness, fatigue and less energy. Balancing these foods with protein and/or healthy fat will make a difference. For example, enjoy a sweet and starchy yam with soy-free Earth Balance®, olive, coconut or flax oil.

❋ To rule out anemia, have your iron and ferritin levels checked. *Ferritin is a measure of your store of iron. Low iron levels can also cause sugar/sweet cravings.*

BREASTFEEDING:

(in addition to the other items noted above)

❋ Choosing small, frequent snacks and meals power-packed with nutrients can combat your cravings. The smoothies and bon bons in this book are excellent choices for alkalinizing your system and providing you with calcium and other important nutrients to satisfy your appetite. If you find in the pre-pregnancy stage that you are sensitive to nuts, you can make most of these recipes by substituting seeds for nuts. *(See the* List of Allergen-Free Recipes *on pages 331-337 to determine which recipes are suitable for your specific needs.)*

❋ Drinking filtered water during every 24-hour period will not only help you maintain your milk supply and prevent dehydration, but it will also minimize your sugar cravings.

❋ To reduce your cravings, make sure your daily meals and snacks contain adequate amounts of protein.

Along with the recommendations above, I advise that you and your spouse/partner make time to discuss your beliefs about sugar and food choices in reference to raising your children. There are no right and wrong answers, however, having an understanding ahead of time helps you both remain committed to eating healthy for yourselves and for your children. Discussing these details in advance creates a flowing dynamic around family mealtimes and provides a smoother transition when solid foods are incorporated into your children's diets.

What remains important is being honest about your relationship to sweets and food. Children don't drive themselves to a fast food restaurant. They can't learn to eat certain foods if those foods aren't a part of your household or lifestyle. With childhood obesity and juvenile diabetes on the rise, discussing the sugar topic could be a priority on your list of projects to complete before the baby arrives.

Though food choices will remain an ongoing topic of discussion as your child grows and develops, creating a "healthy food foundation" at the beginning is very important. From the beginning, with those first smiles, children learn from you and begin imitating you. Our ability to respond (our "responsibility") to their changing needs becomes vital. Eating is an activity of pleasure that we choose at least three times a day. Choosing nourishing and true "growing food" (food that helps your children to grow in healthy ways) has implications beyond measure.

Most people agree that they want what is "best" for their child/ren. Finding your *sweetness* within will also help you guide your child in finding his/her *sweetness*.

> The most important ingredient is love. We eat love when we choose nutrient-dense, healthy, non-manufactured foods for ourselves and our families.

You can create healthy boundaries around healthy foods while eating treats, enjoying food, and creating space for your children to shine their unique light on the world.

Just as your new baby will take baby steps in his/her development, I recommend the same for you and your partner. For more information about planning for a healthy pregnancy, including nutrient needs, fish recommendations, vitamins and supplements, go to *www.vigdorhess.com*.

(For more ideas, see Chapter 3: Exploring the Reasons Behind the Reach *on pages 17-20.)*

Letting go of the "what ifs" (if = I fail) and replacing them with "what is" (is = I succeed) can be a powerful and wondrous experience..

CHAPTER 5:

Sugar SAD

Sugar's Effects on Moods, Emotions and Weight

So long as sugar is on the tongue, you feel the sweetness in taste.
Similarly, so long as the heart has love, peace and devotion,
you feel the bliss.

-Sri Sathya Sai Baba

Sugar and sweeteners can have numerous deleterious effects on our health and our appetites. Sugar affects your mood, emotions and weight. The ingestion of excess sugar can result in a roller coaster of blood sugar ebbs and flows. Contrary to what you might think, this is not the result of poor willpower. Rather, it relates to the physiological processing of sugar in our bodies. Standard or low-calorie diets strongly influence and affect thyroid health, weight fluctuations, and psychological health. "Sugar SAD" is my definition. It is a combination of the "standard American diet" and the common "sadness" and self-judgment that many people experience after eating sugar.

Sugar consumption, along with other factors, has resulted in our growing obesity epidemic and a host of many other health concerns. The invention of low-calorie and artificial sweeteners has also contributed to this new state of sugar addiction and "Sugar SAD". Ingredients added to our food supply (e.g. GMO corn/soy, pesticides, antibiotics, food dyes, excitotoxins, certain preservatives, etc.) have also contributed to this condition.

When you eat carbohydrate foods, your pancreas secretes a hormone called insulin. Insulin removes the sugar from the blood and moves it to the muscles, organs, brain, tissues and the rest of the nervous system where blood sugar can provide energy. After "filtering" to the body systems, the insulin signals the liver to store some sugar for quick energy. The remaining excess sugar is stored as fat.

Complex carbohydrates (e.g. whole grains, legumes, vegetables) and energy released from fat cells provide our body with the amount of sugar needed to maintain homeostasis without the addition of any additional sugar. In this balanced relationship with sugar, serotonin, a brain chemical, is released, signaling satiety and a message to stop eating. More often, excess sugar consumption compromises the body systems, resulting in more sugar cravings, mood swings, weight gain, blood sugar imbalances (e.g. diabetes, hypo/hyperglycemia), a "lull" in energy, decreased immunity and even depressed emotions. Sugar and processed carbohydrates (e.g. white flour, white sugar, "boxed" foods) cause the body to over-secrete insulin.

Some people respond to this excess insulin by "letting" their muscles and organs take in more sugar, causing blood sugar levels to drop quickly. Adrenaline, the "fight or flight" hormone, may be released when the body recognizes low blood sugar. Though it can provide a helpful boost of energy in emergency situations, adrenaline may cause a person to become hyperactive, unfocused and frenzied. Other people have a different response to the deluge of insulin. Their bodies choose not to take in the extra insulin and become insulin-resistant. The blood sugar fuel must go somewhere and is often stored in the fat cells, causing weight gain and an undernourished body.

In both of these examples, the serotonin response is compromised, leaving the person feeling unsatisfied and craving more sugar. In addition, the hormone leptin is effected by both the quantity and form of carbohydrate eaten (e.g. processed and fatty carbohydrates versus slow-sustaining complex carbohydrates). Hence the addictive sugar cycle strongly effects most people and also contributes to a variety of metabolic disorders. This cycle and the increase in sugar ingestion has "SADly" become a mainstay of the Standard American Diet (SAD). What many people consider a lack of willpower is actually a physiological opiate reaction to eating out of alignment with our body's natural needs. This is good news because it can be changed.

Overeating and consuming foods with a high glycemic index may contribute to weight gain. The glycemic index (GI) measures the effect of glucose on blood sugar. Because sweeteners other than glucose effect blood sugar, glycemic index is not the only determinant in assessing your bodies' ability to assimilate sugar or other sweeteners. Also, due to the fact that foods with varying forms of sugar (e.g. sucrose, fructose, glucose) respond and metabolize differently, I do not recommend relying on GI as an accurate predictor. It is important to examine your responses to eating certain fruits and foods sweetened with alternative sweeteners.

There are multiple reasons why we crave sugar and sweets. Often, physiological imbalances cause cravings, resulting in a variety of symptoms such as low blood sugar, fatigue, hormone-related low serotonin levels, and depression. Cravings can also be the result of hormonal imbalances, low adrenal function, food allergies, minimal protein intake, low-fat diets and inflammation. Many of these symptoms are compounded by choices people make because they want to "eat healthy." What is healthy for one may not be for another. We are all unique and have specific metabolic types.

This concept may be most easily understood in this example: Perhaps a diet that worked well for a friend did not work for you; you felt worse, your cravings persisted, and you blamed yourself for your lack of willpower. This is because different people assimilate the same fuel in different ways because of individual differences in blood sugar fluctuations, metabolic and adrenal conditions, and levels of insulin resistance.

Learning more about your body's physiological responses to sugar and artificial sweeteners is important. It is possible to reduce and eliminate "Sugar SAD" from your life. You may wish to start noticing what leads you to reach for a sweet item (e.g. fatigue, sadness, boredom, "a time out," stress, etc.). Having the courage to acknowledge these personal triggers can provide enormous change in your "sweetness journey".

In addition to looking into your personal emotional cues, here are a few additional tips for minimizing sugar addiction:

1. Every day, drink an adequate amount of filtered water (e.g. about 75 ounces of water for every 150 pounds of body weight).

2. Eat more high-quality protein for your unique metabolic needs.

3. Exercise for 30 minutes at least three times per week.

4. Eliminate soda and sports drinks.

5. Reduce or eliminate consumption of caffeinated items like coffee, tea, soda and chocolate.

6. Eliminate from your diet all artificial sweeteners and low-fat and fat-free foods that contain artificial sweeteners. Replace them with whole foods and alternative sweeteners (in moderation).

7. Reduce your intake of processed, heated and chemically-treated sodium (e.g. canned and packaged foods, iodized salt, table salt). Instead, consider obtaining your sodium from mineral-rich and pollutant-free sources such as sea salt, Himalayan crystal salt, seaweeds or cultured vegetables.

    The Food and Drug Administration recommends 2400mg or less sodium per day. *Sodium requirements differ for individuals diagnosed with certain diseases.* Check nutritional information labels to ensure that any processed food you consume contains no more than 140mg of sodium per serving.

    Salt intake affects sugar cravings. Salt is a more contractive (or yang) food, while sugar and sweets are more expansive in nature (or yin). If you have a natural desire for balance, consuming too much salt will trigger your sweet tooth and vice versa. Maintaining a healthy balance between these two natural desires will help control your cravings in either direction.

8. Consider incorporating a green smoothie into your daily diet. For recipe ideas, please see pages 229-242. For a basic green smoothie, choose your favorite fruit, dairy-free milk or filtered water, and greens you like (e.g. Romaine lettuce, spinach, kale, collards, parsley, etc.) Add as many greens as you can - so you still enjoy the taste of the smoothie. Work towards having a quart or more of smoothie a day. Add more greens on a regular basis (up to a bunch or more per day per person).

9. Breathing and mindfulness help us slow down and connect to our natural state of being: our essence and desires. Even taking three deep belly breaths or mindfully repeating a personal mantra or personal positive affirmation is like pushing a re-set button.

10. Make time every day to breathe fresh air. Going outside in all kinds of weather provides us with nourishment and nutrients to feed our soul.

11. Studies show that every dollar spent on wellness saves three dollars in healthcare costs. Transitioning from highly-sweetened and processed foods to more wholesome choices is an important step.

12. Eating at regular intervals (e.g. every three to four hours) is imperative for balancing blood sugar. Healthy fats and protein sources are two necessary ingredients that help restore blood sugar health.

This book is meant to be a stepping stone for making dietary changes while incorporating superfood nutrients and nutritional support. Included are some important steps for altering your relationship with sugar. Please see the *Appendix and Resources* section on pages 316-317 for more books on this subject. For assistance with putting these steps together and attaining personal health goals, readers may feel free to contact me.

CHAPTER 6

Alkaline

Balance

The place where you are right now, God circled on a map for you.

-Hafiz

Once we digest, absorb and metabolize our food, either an acid or alkaline base/ash is left in the blood. Sugar and artificial sweeteners are among the list contributing to an acidic condition in the body, and they have been linked to a variety of health conditions. The importance of maintaining a more alkaline internal environment to obtain optimal health has been observed and written about extensively. Your specific metabolic type also provides a guideline for determining ways to optimize your health through the food choices you make, while taking into account your specific acidic/alkaline balance.

When choosing to make more conscious steps towards optimizing health, you may consider exploring the benefits of reducing acidic conditions in your body. Choosing to omit the sugar and artificial sweeteners in your diet is a wonderful step towards alkalizing your body.

Many foods have been categorized as alkaline, neutral or acidic. As a general guideline, foods that leave a more acidic residue in the body after digestion include grains, meat, dairy, fish, salt, sugar, artificial sweeteners, white and refined foods and flours, and many over-the-counter medications. Nuts can also be an acid-forming food, so with the recipes containing nuts in *Sweetness Without Sugar*, I have mentioned ways to reduce the possibility of creating an acidic state in the body. Some ideas include soaking or sprouting nuts and seeds, or purchasing pre-soaked/pre-sprouted varieties. Those without almond sensitivities can enjoy eating almonds (in conservative amounts). This nut has an alkalizing effect on most people.

Having a more acidic condition in the body can contribute to mineral loss, which can create negative symptoms and exacerbate existing conditions. A normal pH for our blood is between 7.35 and 7.45. Acidic pH is below 7.0 and alkaline pH is above 7.0. Like any continuum, it is beneficial to have a balance. Current scientific research discusses many common links between diet and disease. Some examples include: obesity and diabetes, high cholesterol and hypertension, and high cholesterol and heart disease. It is vital to recognize that excess sugar consumption, toxic and environmental stress, unwise food choices, inflammation and an imbalance in a person's pH can all severely impact a person's health.

With all of these examples, a change in dietary factors can improve symptoms. Incorporating more alkaline foods into the diet can improve conditions such as headaches, GERD, frequent colds and flu, fatigue and low energy.

Stevia is an alkalizing alternative sweetener. Sweeteners such as whole maple syrup or unsulphured molasses can also create a more alkaline balance. Acidifying foods include refined sugar, corn syrup, brown sugar, artificial sweeteners, artificially-sweetened products, commercial maple syrup (which often contains corn syrup and other sweeteners), commercial fruit juices and sulphured molasses. Most people benefit from consuming more alkalizing foods. Always consider your personal metabolic type when selecting the right sweeteners for you.

Even when choosing healthy foods, more is not necessarily better. Variety is an important key. Aiming for a shift toward a more alkaline system is a goal that can be reached in steps. Omitting sugar and artificial sweeteners can have a dramatic effect on one's acid/alkaline balance, and in so doing, open the door for future positive health changes.

A positive goal would be to consume a diet consisting of 60% alkaline-forming foods and 40% acid-forming foods, working toward an 80/20 ratio, respectively. For a handout delineating some of these food categories, please feel free to contact me. If you would like to read more on this subject, I suggest William Wolcott's *The Metabolic Typing Diet*.

CHAPTER 7:

Essential

Fatty Acids

*Man cannot discover new oceans unless he has the courage
to lose sight of the shore.*

-Andre Gide

Essential fatty acids (EFAs), otherwise known as omega 3 (EPA/DHA) and omega 6 (Linoleic and GLA oils), are essential to human health. Ground flax seed, when used as an egg replacer (as in many recipes included in this book), adds more fiber and essential fatty acids into your diet. Research indicates that flax seeds, when heated, tend to break down. Their chemical structure is twisted and changed, rendering heated flax unhealthful to the body, so cooking with flax seed oil is not advised. In baking, however, flax seeds are protected from the light and oxygen, and they remain at a safe temperature for consumption.

In nutritional literature, nutrients are called "essential" because your body cannot make them; you must get them from your diet or from nutritional supplements. Experts agree that a diet deficient in EFAs is hazardous to your health. Your body is made up of one trillion cells, and every cell needs EFAs for energy and to make cell walls. EFAs make up 50% of the gray matter in the human brain. The brain needs fat to help to lubricate neurotransmitters.

EFAs have been shown to offer many additional benefits, such as:

❀ Hormone and immune system function optimization

❀ Reduced inflammation and pain

❀ Production of hormones

❋ Support for clearer thinking

❋ Eyesight and color perception improvement

❋ Support for healthier skin (including firmer, smoother, improved tone and color)

❋ Reduction or elimination of food allergies/sensitivities

❋ Help with a cycle of bingeing and/or an addictive need for food

❋ Increased fat metabolism

❋ Increased resistance to cold weather

❋ Improved digestive tract functioning (e.g. the potential for less gas, constipation and other disorders)

❋ Stronger cardiovascular system (research has addressed many related topics such as atherosclerosis, blood platelets, blood pressure and cholesterol)

The general and minimum recommendation for EFA supplementation is one teaspoon of omega 3 oil per day for each thirty-five to fifty pounds of body weight. A more conservative dosage of omega 3 oil is to consume 300 mg (0.3g) combined EPA/DHA for every ten pounds of body weight. Although omega 6 oil is also essential, it is more readily found in our food supply and most people regularly consume high amounts of omega 6. *Check with your pediatrician or healthcare provider for recommendations for infants and children, as they are more specific.*

It is important to consider the ratio of omega 3 to omega 6 oil one consumes when supplementing these nutrients. Research has shown that varying ratios are ideal for treating different health conditions when one's total fat intake (in addition to omega oils) must be optimized. Recommendations can be provided by your healthcare provider.

Most people would benefit from increasing their intake of omega 3 oils and reducing their intake of omega 6 oils. Consuming a healthy omega 6 oil (such as GLA) will help balance a higher dosage of omega 3 oil. To personalize recommendations, testing is available through several laboratories (e.g. Genova Diagnostics® and Metametrix™ Clinical Laboratory). The results will indicate your unique needs.

Food Sources of Omega 6 Fatty Acids

❈ *Arachidonic Acid (AA or ARA)*: some animal products (including meat) and peanut oil *(not recommended due to aflatoxins found in peanuts). Some research indicates that Arachidic Acid (not Arachidonic Acid) is present in peanuts. Arachidic Acid is a long-chain saturated fat.*

❈ *Gamma-linolenic Acid (GLA)*: evening primrose oil, borage oil, black currant seed oil and spirulina powder.

❈ *Linoleic Acid (LA)*: sesame seeds, pumpkin seeds, hempseed, flax seed, many nuts and most vegetable oils, especially safflower and sunflower oils.[*]

Food Sources of Omega 3 Fatty Acids

❈ *Alpha-linolenic Acid (ALA or LNA)*: flax seed, hempseed, pumpkin seeds, walnuts, dark green leafy vegetables, chia seeds, kukui (candlenut), canola oil and soy.

❈ *Eicosapentaenoic Acid (EPA) and Docosahexaenoic Acid (DHA)*: salmon, trout, krill, mackerel and sardines. *The vegan source is made from microalgae.*

❈ *Stearidonic Acid (SDA)*: black currant seeds and some non-commercialized wild seeds.

Vegan Sources Of Omega 3 Oils

❈ Chia seeds

❈ DHA or microalgae supplements such as Tachyon™, Crystal Manna™ or E3Live™ [**]

---

[*] *Many of the recipes included in this book incorporate walnut or sunflower oil. Sunflower oil is high in omega 6 and may be refined (if in a high-heat form), and can be substituted with a melted coconut oil or walnut oil.*

[**] *Obtain recommendations and dosage from a qualified registered dietitian (RD) and/or health practitioner.*

Vegan Sources Of Omega 3 Oils (continued)

❁ Flax oil

❁ Flax seed, whole or ground

❁ Hemp oil

❁ Hempseed

❁ Pumpkin seeds, raw

❁ Sesame seeds, raw

❁ Walnuts, raw

Flax Oil and Flax Seed

Flax seeds contain an abundance of omega 3 oil, B vitamins, magnesium, phosphorus and other micronutrients. The seeds are also high in dietary fiber and have been shown to help stabilize blood sugar levels. Buying fresh flax seeds and grinding them to use within a few days can prevent rancidity and provide a tasty way to obtain this important nutrient. Store flax oil and seeds in the refrigerator for short-term use, and in the freezer for long-term use. Be sure to consume the products by the expiration date. (If they have a strong smell or taste, they may be rancid.) Flax oil is also available for supplementation in pill/capsule form, however, to reach the dosages commonly recommended, many pills are required.

Specific suggestions regarding consumption of omega oil sources are best determined by your healthcare practitioner. It is important to choose oils from uncontaminated sources because supplements often contain unnecessary fillers.

Once you achieve a healthier omega oil balance, consuming flax in addition to other healthy omega 3 oils will help prevent an omega 6 deficiency. Though many add omega oils to their diets due to omega 3 deficiencies, they often have an excess of omega 6 as a result of consuming processed foods and oils. After a year or two of consuming flax oil, omega 6 levels will decrease. Incorporating other omega oils (from the above list) into your diet will help maintain an optimal balance.

Coconut Oil

Coconut oil, though not an omega 3 or 6 oil, is included in many of the recipes in this book. Some of the benefits of coconut oil include: the nutrient value of medium-chain fatty acids (found in human breast milk); its anti-microbial, anti-viral, anti-fungal properties; high amounts of lauric acid; and stability with high heat. Although a saturated fat, coconut oil is not hydrogenated. Other plant-based, non-hydrogenated saturated fats include palm oil and cocoa butter*. The amount of lauric acid in coconut oil differs between brands and production quality standards. Coconut oil contains no protein, carbohydrates, sugar or cholesterol and it helps to break up and metabolize accumulated fats.

There are differences between coconut oils. Some are labeled as virgin, others, refined. Virgin coconut oils are made from fresh coconuts and have a much stronger and distinct taste, smell and texture. Most use some heat in the processing, whereas raw oils do not and their shelf life may be shorter. Refined coconut oils are produced from the "meat" of the coconut. This meat, or copra, is often smoke-, sun- or kiln-dried, which can result in impurities and mycotoxins (unhealthy toxins produced by fungi). These impurities may be removed by bleaching, deodorizing and chemical processing. To purchase the highest quality coconut oil, look for companies that make products from virgin coconuts.

To purchase omega 3 oils of the highest quality, choose oils with these features**:

- ❀ Bottled in opaque, glass or earthen containers
- ❀ Mechanically-pressed (vs. chemically-pressed with the use of solvents)
- ❀ Processed below 118°F
- ❀ Processed excluding light and air
- ❀ Processed without toxic solvents
- ❀ Unrefined and unheated
- ❀ Made from pesticide-free seeds

---

*   *Avoid products when the food label states hydrogenated palm oil or cocoa butter. Though naturally unhydrogenated, processing and manufacturing may change their structure.*
**   *Purchasing less processed foods and using the savings toward the purchase of high-quality oils will be of great benefit to you.*

To purchase other oils of the highest quality, choose oils with these features*:

❋ Mechanically-pressed oils.

❋ Virgin, extra virgin or unrefined varieties (to avoid possible processing with other oils, solvents and chemicals).**

❋ Store oils in a cool, dry place (or keep in the refrigerator or freezer). This helps preserve freshness, prevent rancidity and optimizes the benefits of these oils.

❋ Check expiration dates to ensure freshness.

❋ Use oils within three to six weeks after opening.

❋ Avoid hydrogenated oils and those containing trans-fatty acids.

❋ Purchase organic and pesticide-free seed oils.

To improve your overall health and fat balance, avoid these fats:

❋ Hydrogenated and partially-hydrogenated fats

❋ Shortening

❋ Trans fatty acids

❋ Peanut*** and cottonseed*** oils

❋ Margarine

❋ Corn oil***

❋ Soy oil***

❋ Canola oil***

---

* Purchasing less processed foods and using the savings toward the purchase of high-quality oils will be of great benefit to you.

** High-quality virgin, extra virgin and unrefined olive or other oils should be clearly labeled. Olive oil does not contain omega oils, however, it is a monosaturated fat that is healthy and stable.

*** Aflatoxins may be found in peanuts. Corn, soy, canola and cotton are the most genetically-modified crops on the market today.

CHAPTER 8:

Corn,

Corn Sugar and
High Fructose Corn Syrup

I will act as if what I do makes a difference.
-William James

When the average person increases his/her sugar intake, he/she also increases his/her consumption of fructose (from corn syrup or corn sugar), perhaps without realizing it. In the early '80's, amid our growing obesity epidemic, the average annual consumption of sucrose was 84 pounds. The average annual consumption of fructose was 39 pounds. In the early '90's, these figures changed to 66 and 83 pounds, respectively. After years of talking with people, and witnessing the economic trends related to the purchase and consumption of sugar, I have noticed a pattern of misunderstanding. Many people believe that eating sugar-free foods is one key to better health. This belief causes them to consume more fruit sugar, or in many cases, fructose (in the form of high fructose corn syrup, corn syrup, agave or other manufactured sweeteners). From these recent statistics, it is easy to note that the significant reduction in sucrose consumption and increase in fructose consumption have not reduced the cases of obesity or diabetes.

Although fructose is abundant in nature through a wide variety of fruits, the most common form is found in high fructose corn syrup (HFCS), which also contains glucose. HFCS is now prevalent in our food supply. The corn used to make HCFS is subsidized by the government and genetically-modified (to reduce costs). Due to high demand, corn manufacturing has caused more soil erosion and depletion of soil nutrients than any other crop.

The natural form of fructose is different from HCFS. When eating fruit, we receive fiber and other nutrients, which slow absorption of the sugar. On the other hand, when we drink soft drinks and juices containing corn syrup made from genetically-modified corn, we absorb and metabolize the sweetener more quickly.

In the Singapore Chinese Health Study, which studied 60,000 men and women over a period of fourteen years, researchers found that people who drank two or more sweetened soft drinks (12 ounces each) per week had a higher risk of pancreatic cancer. Though the research was not controlled for other adverse health and dietary habits, the results remain startling.

Fructose, like sucrose, spikes blood sugar but does not stimulate insulin secretion. Instead, fructose is metabolized by the liver so foods with higher fructose may not register high on the glycemic index. Current research suggests this bodily response (along with leptin production) affects appetite regulation because both insulin and leptin are hormones that help the body self-regulate. Consequently, fructose may be converted into fat more quickly than other sugars. When these hormones are out of balance, they greatly effect ones' cravings, weight fluctuations and mood. This reality creates a common cycle for people struggling with sugar addiction, weight issues and a host of common diseases. If you are interested in more details about how fructose is metabolized in your body, see *Sugar: The Bitter Truth* by Dr. Robert Lustig, UCSF Professor of Pediatrics in the Division of Endocrinology: *http://www.youtube.com/watch?v=dBnniua6-oM.*

A high intake of fructose may also deplete the body's supply of magnesium and other necessary minerals, contribute to a more acidic internal environment and cause insulin resistance. Fructose has been shown to inhibit copper metabolism, resulting in a reduction of our bodies' ability to produce elastin and collagen. It can also lead to other health concerns. Many manufacturers continue to use mercury-contaminated sodium hydroxide during production of HFCS. Though the quantities of mercury found during production were less than the amount of mercury found in dental fillings, mercury fillings can be a significant contributor to increased mercury toxicity and associated health hazards.

Recent articles printed in *Advertising Age* (August 20, 2009) and *Crain's Chicago Business* (August 24, 2009) reported that several large manufacturers including Kraft Foods, Con Agra, PepsiCo, Starbucks and Snapple removed HFCS from some of their products. This was largely due to consumer demand and the manufacturers' desires to transition away from using HFCS in their products.

Although many of the reformulated foods and drinks include variations of cane sugar (a sugar I don't recommend for consumption in most cases), I mention this recent article to demonstrate that our choices as consumers can make a difference in changing products that are sold.

> When we choose products containing wholesome sweeteners (and other healthy, clearly-labeled, non genetically-modified ingredients), we can directly influence the items available in our food supply.

There has been recent speculation that certain brands of processed agave syrup have been "watered down" with corn syrup in order to lower costs. Similarly, some brands are suspected to contain pesticides. In addition to fruit, fructose-rich liquids like honey and agave nectar may cause symptoms associated with sensitivities.

Fructose comes in many forms such as fruit, high fructose corn syrup, agave nectar and honey. The deleterious effects of fructose consumption are becoming more well-known with current research. Some metabolic responses are based on the form of the fructose, while others may indicate a sensitivity to fructose in any form.

Current research on this topic discusses uric acid levels as a marker for fructose sensitivity and/or toxicity. The safest range for uric acid has been shown to be between 3 and 5.5 milligrams per deciliter (mg/dl) with more specific recommendations including a goal of 4 mg/dl for men and 3.5 mg/dl for women. If, upon testing, your serum uric acid levels are high, you may be more sensitive to fructose and may wish to retest after removing corn syrup, agave and fruit drinks from your diet. If your levels are still high (and you consume a lot of fresh fruit), I agree with the current medical recommendations to consider lowering your fruit consumption until you optimize your uric acid levels. In a June 2010 article in his *Natural Health Newsletter*, Dr. Joseph Mercola has included a helpful chart listing the uric acid levels in a variety of fruits. (*See www.articles.mercola.com for more information.*) Please see my recommendations on pages 92-95 for more on fructose-based sweeteners.

After conducting research, experiencing my own "sweet journey" and working with many people effected by problems associated with eating certain foods, I recommend individual approaches to healing based on one's unique body chemistry, health concerns, food sensitivities and family histories. I strongly recommend avoiding high-fructose corn syrup and consuming only non-GMO organic corn and/or corn products.[*]

Every person has a unique body chemistry and metabolic type. Consequently, different people can react to the same food or sweeteners in different ways, and because of this, overconsumption is not recommended. Since products and ingredients change, I encourage you to contact a product manufacturer if you have questions about whether the product will meet your needs.

Foods Containing Corn or Corn Derivatives

Although many people think the only sweetener containing corn is high fructose corn syrup, in fact, a great number of sweeteners are derived from corn. Among these sweeteners are sorbitol, dextrose, erythritol and maltodextrin. As of this writing, corn, like soy, is one of the most genetically-modified foods in the food supply. Corn syrup is added to many popular products such as maple syrup, "convenience" foods and other snacks. Corn has also been shown to contain twenty-five mycotoxic fungi (unhealthy toxins produced by fungi). Consider purchasing products made by companies that grow corn using organic farming methods (without pesticides or herbicides). Certified organic foods are grown without genetically-modified ingredients.

It is also important to remember that your meat and poultry may contain corn because it is often a component of the cattle feed. You may wish to check with your local farmers and ask that grass-fed sources be carried in your local grocery store. Recent research has shown that corn grains may (in some cases) be contaminated by wheat or grains containing gluten. This is important information for people with celiac disease or for those who choose to omit wheat and/or gluten from their diets.

---

[*] *Moldy corn has been shown to contain aflatoxin, a known carcinogen. Corn plants are also commonly fertilized with ammonium nitrate from fossil fuels, contributing to compromised human and environmental health.*

Here is a list of foods that may contain corn or corn derivatives:

- Acetic acid
- Alcohol (whiskey, bourbon, American wines, ale, beer, gin)
- Alpha tocopherol
- Artificial flavorings
- Artificial sweeteners
- Ascorbates
- Ascorbic acid
- Aspirin
- Astaxanthin
- Bacon
- Baked beans
- Bakery products
- Baking powder (see *page 108*)
- Barbecue sauce
- Barley malt
- Biscuit mix
- Biscuits
- Bleached flour
- Blended sugar, sugaridextrose
- Bread
- Brown sugaridextrose
- Cake
- Cake mix
- Calcium citrate
- Calcium fumarate
- Calcium gluconate
- Calcium lactate
- Calcium magnesium acetate
- Calcium stearate
- Calcium stearoyl lactylate
- Candied FruitSource™
- Candy
- Caramel
- Caramel coloring
- Carbonated beverages
- Carbonmethylcellulose sodium
- Carob (check labels)
- Cellulose microcrystalline
- Cellulose, methyl
- Cellulose, powdered
- Cereals, especially pre-sweetened
- Cetearyl glucoside
- Cheese, imitation and non-dairy
- Choline chloride
- Citric acid
- Citrus cloud emulsion (CCS)
- Coffee creamers/ whiteners
- Condiments
- Confectioner's sugar
- Cookies
- Corn
- Corn alcohol
- Corn chips
- Corn flakes
- Corn flour
- Corn oil
- Corn sugar
- Corn sweeteners
- Corn syrup
- Corn syrup solids
- Cornmeal
- Cornstarch (also found in medications)
- Cow's milk (from corn-fed cows)
- Crystalline dextrose
- Crystalline fructose
- Custard
- Cyclodextrin
- Dextrates
- Dextrin
- Dextrose
- d-Gluconic acid
- Doughnuts
- Drying agent
- Equal®
- Erythorbic acid
- Erythritol
- Ethanol
- Ethylcellulose
- Ethylene
- Food starch
- Frozen desserts
- Fructose
- Fruit juice, concentrated
- Fruit juices
- Fumaric acid
- Glucose

continued

- Glucose syrup (for diabetes tests and intravenous applications)
- Glutamate
- Gluten feed/meal
- Glycerides
- Glycerin
- Glycerol
- Golden syrup
- Graham crackers
- Gravy
- Grits
- High-fructose corn syrup (HFCS)
- Hominy
- Honey (some brands contain corn)
- Hydrolyzed corn
- Hydrolyzed corn protein
- Hydroxypropyl methylcellulose
- Hydroxypropyl methylcellulose pthalate (HPMCP)
- Iced tea (canned or bottled)
- Inositol
- Instant coffee
- Invert sugar
- Invert syrup or sugaridextrose
- Iodized salt
- Jam
- Jelly
- Juice drinks (canned or bottled)
- Ketchup
- Lactate
- Lactic acid
- Latin foods
- Lauryl glucoside
- Lecithin
- Linoleic acid
- Lozenges
- Lysine
- Magnesium fumarate
- Maize
- Malic acid
- Malonic acid
- Malt
- Malt extract
- Malt syrup
- Maltitol
- Maltodextrin
- Maltol
- Maltose
- Mannitol
- Margarine
- Methyl gluceth
- Methyl glucose
- Methyl glucoside
- Methylcellulose
- Mexican foods
- Microcrystaline cellulose
- Modified food starch
- Molasses (some brands)
- Mono and diglycerides
- Monosodium glutamate (MSG)
- Nachos
- Nondairy creamers
- Olestra®
- Olean®
- Pancake mix
- Pancake syrup
- Pancakes
- Peanut butter (Jiff®, Peter Pan® and others)
- Pickle relish
- Pickles, sweeteners
- Pie filling
- Polenta
- Polysorbates (Polysorbate 80®)
- Popcorn
- Powdered sugar
- Processed meats
- Pudding
- Saccharin
- Salad dressing
- Sauces
- Semolina
- Sherbet
- Soda
- Sodium citrate
- Soft drinks
- Sorghum (some brands are mixed with corn)
- Sorbic acid
- Sorbitol
- Soup
- Spaghetti sauce

continued

- Splenda®
- Succotash
- Sucrose
- Sugar (if not identified as cane or beet)
- Sweet & Low®
- Syrup
- Threonine
- Tocopherol (Vitamin E)
- Toothpastes
- Tortillas
- Treacle
- Triethyl citrate
- Unmodified starch
- Vanilla extract
- Vanilla flavoring
- Vanilla, natural flavoring
- Vanillin
- Vegetable gum
- Vegetable oil
- Vegetable shortening
- Vegetable starch
- Vegetables, frozen, mixed
- Vinegar, distilled white
- Vinyl acetate
- Vitamin C and Vitamin E
- Vitamins and supplements
- Waffles
- Xanthan gum
- Xylitol (unless from birch source)
- Yeast
- Yogurt, dairy or soy
- Zea mays
- Zein

CHAPTER 9:

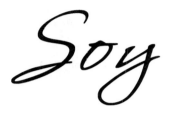

You gain strength, courage and confidence by every experience in which you really stop to look fear in the face.
-Eleanor Roosevelt

In recent years much has been written about soy. I've chosen to include this chapter since many soy products on the market also contain sugar. Also, with the increase in production and consumption of soy products, many people have become aware of their sensitivities to soy foods.

Many baked products or vegan sweets are made with soy products. Although some of the recipes included in this book contain soy, I recommend choosing soy products based on individual needs, family history, intuition and current research. Like many other health quests, for every positive recommendation to incorporate soy into one's diet, there is an opposing view, both generally supported with some sort of research.

As other trends in our society, looking for the "magic pill" has led some people to increase the amount of soy in their diet. Upon learning of the benefits of soy, more manufacturers began making products including soy and adding the recently-researched health benefits and "buzz words" to their food labels.

Soy has been added to a large percentage of our current food supply ranging from soy lecithin to isolated soy protein, resulting in hundreds of millions of dollars of revenue for those selling soy products per year. Similar to the "fat-free craze" or high-protein fad diets, the incorporation of soy also became a pseudo-"diet craze." The research on the benefits of soy most commonly refers to the whole form of soy, rather than genetically-modified soybeans or manufactured soy foods sprayed with toxic chemicals (found in non-organic soy and soy products). Many prepared soy foods also contain both wheat and gluten.

As a dietitian and nutritionist as well as a consumer, I know it can be murky to learn the truth about what choice is best for any one individual. My role is to offer an opinion based on the most current research and allow each individual to decide for her/himself. With my emphasis on whole foods nutrition, I believe in making the distinction between a wholesome choice and a manufactured or "doctored up" version.

If you are incorporating soy into your diet, it's best to choose organic soy sources. Spending additional money on organic soy will likely be less expensive than meats and many other packaged and "convenience" foods. Certified organic foods are grown without genetically-modified ingredients.

Some questions to ask yourself when making the decision about whether soy is right for you:

1. Does the soy product you consume (or want to consume) use whole soy foods? Or does it contain soy isolates or manufactured items containing soy? I recommend eating only whole or fermented soy foods. See page 52 for a more detailed list of my recommendations. *If the ingredients listed on the soy food label are unrecognizable, sound particularly scientific or are hard to pronounce, manufactured soy is often the main ingredient.*

2. How does your body respond to eating food containing soy ingredients?

3. Do you have a family history of cancer? Do any women in your family have an estrogen-positive (ER+) form of breast cancer? If the answer is "yes", and you are a woman, then I recommend you avoid soy products.

4. How strong is your immune system at this time? (e.g. Do you get sick frequently? Are you living with chronic disease? How is your thyroid health?)

Here are some additional questions for families deciding whether to incorporate soy into their family's diet:

1. Are you preparing for conception? Diets high in soy, in some instances, have been linked with infertility.

2. Are you pregnant and/or breastfeeding? If you consume high amounts of soy (4-5 times per week) and you or your baby experience a lot of gas or bloating, reducing your intake may be helpful.

3. How old are your children? Have you already introduced soy into their diet? If so, at what age, in what form and at what frequency? If you haven't already fed soy to your baby, I recommend waiting until they are 2 or older, which will give their immune systems time to mature. If you choose to feed soy to your children, I suggest offering them only organic, fermented forms of soy. Occasionally, they can enjoy sprouted soy products.

4. Have your children been vaccinated? If so, at what age? Vaccinations directly affect our immune systems. Because soy is often listed as one of the foods that can cause sensitivities (related to our immune system function), as mentioned in question #3, I recommend waiting until children are 2 years of age or older before introducing soy into their diets.

5. Are you feeding your children a vegan diet? If so, I recommend obtaining protein and nutrients from sources other than soy. Also, when incorporating soy foods for children, I recommend including only whole food sources of organic soy (see question #3).

If you enjoy reading medical research and articles about the benefits and drawbacks of consuming soy products, here are some questions you may wish to ask yourself after you read the articles. Answers to these questions may help you discern how the findings may apply to your unique situation:

1. In the article, was the testing performed on humans or animals or both? Though results from research performed on animals are frequently compared with that of humans, this is not always the case. Look for research performed on humans.

2. In the study, how much soy did participants consume (vs. the standard recommendation of 2-3 servings of soy per week)? Did participants consume high doses of supplements only? Or did they consume servings of soy food products only? What form of soy was consumed (e.g. fermented soy, soy isolates, organic soy, etc.)?

If high doses of supplements were given to study participants, then results may be very different from results of study participants who ate soy 2-3 times per week. Similarly, if the study participants consumed miso or a fermented soy product, but you ingest tofu, the study results would likely not apply to your situation.

From a research perspective, the healthiest and "safest" soy to incorporate into your diet includes organic versions of fermented soy products such as:

❋ Tempeh

❋ Miso (can also purchase a chickpea miso at some health food stores)

❋ Natto

Organic soy products to use in moderation (if at all), include:

❋ Tamari (this is wheat-free soy sauce) *This is not a fermented soy product.*

❋ Organic tofu (e.g. rotating every 3rd or 4th day)[*] *This is not a fermented soy product.*

Manufactured soy foods to omit or greatly reduce from your diet include:

❋ Soy protein isolates

❋ Hydrolyzed soy protein

❋ Soy oil

❋ Soy protein concentrates

❋ Textured vegetable protein (TVP)

❋ Soy lecithin[**] (unless non-genetically modified - "non-GMO")

❋ Soy supplements or soy ingredients in your supplements

❋ Soy protein powders

❋ Soy milks with added sugar sweeteners (you can make your own with organic soaked and/or sprouted soybeans or choose an unsweetened hemp, almond or rice milk)

---

[*] *I also suggest sprouted organic tofu from Wild Wood Organics™. This is not a fermented product and may or may not be recommended by your healthcare practitioner.*

[**] *Sunflower lecithin is an alternative.*

❋ Soy flour

❋ Any soy foods that are not organic

The soy ingredients in the above list are often found in "protein bars," protein powders, veggie burgers, soy "look- alike" foods such as "chicken fingers", snack foods, baby formula and many other products. For more information, examine the ingredients listed on the labels of the foods you most enjoy.

If you are interested in an article on soy-free vegan living, visit this link:
http://vegkitchen.com/tips/when-soy-annoys.htm

Foods Containing Soy

Like corn, soy is one of the most genetically-modified foods on the market today and is also found in a large percentage of foods in our current food supply. Some of the recipes included in this book contain soy. I always recommend using organic soy products and avoiding genetically-modified soy. Certified organic foods are grown without genetically-modified ingredients.

Over the years, many people have asked my opinion regarding eating soy. Soy has estrogenic properties. As a result of the increased consumer demand for soy, it is not always available in the healthiest form for human consumption. I recommend avoiding and/or limiting soy items that include soy protein isolates, soy protein powders, energy bars containing soy and additional foods for cooking such as soy oil. These forms of soy are generally manufactured and do not contain soy in its whole food form.

It is also important to remember that your meat and poultry may contain soy, as soy is often a component of cattle feed. You may wish to check with your local farmers and ask for grass-fed sources to be carried in your local grocery.

For recommendations about eating soy during pregnancy see Chapter 4 on pages 21-25.

A list of foods that may contain soy is given on the next page:

- Baby foods
- Bakery foods
- Bouillon or stock cubes
- Breads
- Breakfast cereals
- Bulking agents
- Butter substitutes (Earth Balance®* Spectrum®)
- Cake
- Candy
- Canned or packaged soups
- Carob
- Cheese, dairy-free
- Chinese food
- Chocolate
- Cookies
- Cornstarch
- Crackers
- Desserts
- Edamame
- Emulsifier
- Guar gum
- Gum arabic
- Hydrolyzed vegetable protein (HVP)
- Infant formulas
- Lecithin** (from soy or egg)
- Liquid meal replacer
- Margarine
- Meat alternatives (e.g. veggie burgers, tofu dogs, Field Roast®)
- Miso
- Monosodium glutamate (MSG) from soy or wheat
- Muesli
- Non-dairy/dairy-free frozen desserts
- Pies
- Powdered meal replacer
- Protein
- Protein extender
- Salad dressings
- Sauces (Worcestershire, hoisin, teriyaki)
- Seasoned salt
- Shortening
- Shoyu
- Soups
- Soy flour
- Soy nuts
- Soy panthenol
- Soy pasta (some other pastas contain soy)
- Soy protein
- Soy protein isolate or concentrate
- Soy sauce
- Soy sprouts
- Soya
- Soybean
- Soybean oil
- Stabilizer
- Supplements/vitamins
- Tamari
- Tempeh
- Textured soy protein
- Textured vegetable protein (TVP)
- Thickening agents
- Tofu
- Vegetable broth
- Vegetable gum
- Vegetable starch
- Vitamin E

---

*   *Earth Balance® now makes a soy-free version.*
** *Sunflower lecithin is also available.*

CHAPTER 10:

Food

Allergies and Sensitivities

To be yourself in a world that is constantly trying to make you something else is the greatest accomplishment.

-Ralph Waldo Emerson

ood allergies and sensitivities are very common and often under-reported. There are blood and skin tests available that highlight areas of sensitivity. You can find many resources for learning more about how these can effect your digestion, quality of health, and overall life.

Often, when people make major life changes, they may also notice changes in their digestion and assimilation of commonly eaten foods, even foods that have never caused them a negative reaction in the past. If, after removing certain foods from your diet, you still have symptoms, a blood test or further investigation may be a solid next step. Although living with sensitivities may seem limiting, with planning, you will find these suggestions easy to incorporate into your diet, offering you a gift for your long-term health. For helpful resources on this subject, please see the *Appendix and Resource* section on pages 293-317.

It is imperative that we, as consumers, educate ourselves about new products and product ingredients in our food supply. It is especially important that we understand the health implications of the ingredients in some alternative sweeteners. I recently had a nutritional session with someone who mentioned having a reaction to agave. Alternatives may be more wholesome, but they may still cause a reaction in some people. To continue maintaining your health, always insure that the brands of food you purchase contain quality ingredients.

Here are some tips that may be helpful when addressing food sensitivities and/or allergies:

1. Soaking and/or sprouting nuts and seeds helps with digestion and assimilation. See page 134 for a guide for soaking and sprouting.

2. If a family member has a food sensitivity, one option is to incorporate the food on a rotating basis. Check with your healthcare practitioner to learn more about the consequences, risks or symptoms of specific food sensitivities. Also feel free to contact me to discuss your unique needs.

3. Although most people believe food allergies and sensitivities require that a food must be avoided, the goal in prevention and treatment is to teach the body to recognize the food as a friend, rather than an enemy. *If there is an actual anaphylaxis allergy or if celiac sprue has been diagnosed, the food must be avoided. Working with your healthcare practitioners (trained with food allergies) is advised.*

4. People often crave the very things that cause their symptoms. Having examined the results of many food allergy blood tests, I know it is common for people to be highly reactive to many of the foods they eat regularly.

5. Food allergies and sensitivities can result from shifts in a persons' body chemistry (*for more information, see* Chapter 6: Alkaline Balance *on pages 33-34*). They also can result from other conditions such as irritable bowel syndrome and/or leaky gut. By thoroughly examining the whole person (including his/her emotional health), health can be restored and allergies and sensitivities can be minimized or disappear completely.

6. People often notice they become less sensitive to many of their triggers when gluten and dairy are removed from their diets.

7. Evaluate your intake of vitamins and supplements.

8. Drinking adequate amounts of water to prevent dehydration has also been shown to be helpful in minimizing the histamine responses. Here are a few general guidelines for water intake:

   a. Drink half your weight in ounces of water per day (e.g. a 150-lb person should drink 75 oz. of filtered water per day).

   b. For every 50 lbs of your body weight, drink 1 quart of water (e.g. a 150-lb person should drink 3 quarts or 96 oz. of filtered water per day).

   c. If you drink caffeinated beverages, also drink eight additional ounces of water for every eight ounces of caffeinated beverage consumed.

   d. Drink more water during and after exercise: approximately four to six ounces of water per fifteen minutes of cardiovascular exercise.

   e. Consuming adequate amounts of water ensures that urine output is clear.

Though urine may be clear after drinking caffeinated beverages, caffeine actually dehydrates the body.

Foods Containing Dairy Products

If you have a dairy sensitivity or allergy, it is important to understand the sources for your milk and dairy products. If the cows or goats that supply your dairy products have been fed genetically-modified corn and/or soy, your reactions may be related to more than just dairy products. Check with your local farmer about his/her organic practices, or consider buying organic products from sources processed without hormones, antibiotics, or pesticides. Certified organic foods are grown without genetically-modified ingredients.

A list of foods that may contain dairy products is given on the next page:

- Artificial butter flavor
- Baked goods
- Batter-fried foods
- Biscuits
- Breaded foods
- Breads
- Breakfast cereals
- Butter
- Butterfat
- Buttermilk
- Cake
- Candy
- Caramel
- Casein
- Caseinate
- Cheese, all kinds (American, Swiss, etc.)
- Chocolate
- Coated nuts or seeds
- Cookies
- Cottage cheese
- Crackers
- Cream
- Cream cheese
- Cream sauce
- Creamed soups
- Curd
- Custard
- Energy bars

- Evaporated milk
- Feta cheese
- Filled candy bars
- Flavored teas
- Ghee
- Goat cheese*
- Goat yogurt*
- Gravies and/or gravy mixes
- Half and Half®
- High-protein flour
- Hydrosylates (milk protein or protein)
- Ice cream
- Instant potato flakes
- Kefir (unless coconut kefir)
- Kosher symbol "D" or "DE"
- Lactalbumin
- Lactalbumin phosphate
- Lactoglobulin
- Lactose
- Lactulose
- Margarine
- Mashed potatoes
- Milk
- Muesli
- Muffins

- Natural flavoring
- Non-dairy "cheese"
- Non-fat dry milk
- Nougat
- Ovaltine®
- Packaged soups
- Pancakes
- Pasta sauce
- Pies
- Pizza sauce
- Products/ingredients beginning with "lacta-" or "lacto-" (e.g. lactobacillus, etc.)
- Pudding
- Quark
- Rennet casein
- Ricotta
- Rusks
- Salad dressings
- Simplesse®
- Skim milk
- Sour cream
- Soy cheese
- Supplements/vitamins
- Syrups
- Whey
- Whipped toppings
- Yogurt

---

* *People sensitive to products made from cow's milk can sometimes tolerate goat's milk. Please note that some goat's milk products may also contain cow's milk. Read product labels closely and/or check with manufacturers for information.*

Foods Containing Egg or Egg Derivatives

If you are sensitive to eggs, test both the yolks and whites to determine if both cause symptoms for you. Similar to a dairy sensitivity or allergy, it is important to understand the source for your eggs. If the chickens whose eggs you consume have been fed genetically-modified corn and/or soy, your allergic reactions may be related to more than just eggs. Ask your local farmers about how their chickens are raised. Certified organic foods are grown without genetically-modified ingredients. Chickens may be fed foods containing common allergens (e.g. corn or soy).

Here is a list of foods that may contain egg or egg derivatives:

- Albumin
- Avidin
- Baked goods
- Baking mixes
- Batters
- Bearnaise sauce
- Breakfast cereals
- Conalbumin
- Cookies
- Cream fillings
- Custard
- Egg
- Egg-based binding agents
- Egg-based coagulants
- Egg nog
- Egg noodles
- Egg white
- Egg yellow
- Egg yolk
- Emulsifier
- French toast
- Globulin
- Hollandaise sauce
- Ice cream
- Instant Cream of Wheat®
- Instant oatmeal
- Lecithin
- Lemon curd
- Lipovitelin
- Livetin
- Lysozyme
- Malted drinks
- Mayonnaise
- Meringue
- Mousse
- Muffins
- Nougats
- Omelettes
- Ova
- Ovalbumin
- Ovamucin
- Ovo
- Ovomucin
- Ovomucoid
- Ovotransferrin
- Ovovitellin
- Pancakes
- Pavlova mix
- Phosvitin
- Powdered egg
- Protein powders
- Pudding
- Quiche
- Salad dressings
- Sherbet
- Silici albuminate
- Souffles
- Soups
- Spreads for sandwiches
- Tartar sauce
- Tempura
- Vitellin
- Waffles
- Whole egg
- Wines
- Yolk

Foods Containing Gluten

Gluten, the protein found in wheat and products containing wheat, is hidden in many common foods. During baking, the protein makes the final product stick together. Research has shown that when gluten breaks down during digestion, it produces a mild opiate effect. Unfortunately, gluten sensitivity is linked to common diseases such as anemia and osteoporosis. Those who are sensitive to this protein may also report a change in moods and/or cravings (among other symptoms) when gluten is removed from their diets.

Blood tests are available that determine if you or a family member are sensitive to gluten and/or have celiac disease.* The symptoms of this disease can be "silent" in that they may be easily attributable to other conditions such as stress. Celiac is commonly overlooked, although the rates of incidence are on the rise perhaps due to current research and the damaging effects celiac may cause. Some gluten/celiac marker blood tests to ask for may include: HLA-DQ2, HLA-DQ8, tTG-IgA and deaminated gliadin and antigliadin AB. If needed, additional tests are available.

If you have tested negative for celiac disease, gluten intolerance, and wheat intolerance and allergy (IgG and IgE, respectively), but continue to notice symptoms, you may be sensitive to a substance in wheat called wheat germ agglutinin (WGA). This substance is found in high concentrations in both sprouted wheat and whole wheat and can have a variety of adverse effects on the body. To read more about this topic, please see the articles by Sayer Ji noted in the *Bibliography* on pages 319-320. Dr. Gabriel Cousens has also written about research on lectins (sugar-binding proteins) in his book, *Conscious Eating*, and other publications.

On the next page is a list of foods that may contain gluten:

---

*   *If blood test results are inconclusive, gene tests can be used to determine if you have celiac disease.*

- Ale
- Baked beans
- Baking powder
- Barley
- Barley malt
- Beer
- Bread
- Broth with vegetable protein added
- Brown rice syrup (certain brands)
- Bulgur
- Candy
- Caramel
- Cereal
- Chips with seasonings
- Citric acid
- Coffee (some flavored coffees)
- Cornbread
- Couscous
- Dairy foods (some dairy foods frequently contain gluten)
- Dairy-free milks, sweetened with malt
- Dessert mixes (e.g. frosting, cake and pudding mixes)
- Dextrin
- Dried dates dusted with flour
- Durum wheat pasta
- Egg substitute
- Einkorn
- Emergen-C
- Emmer
- Farro
- Flavorings
- Flour
- Flour tortillas or wraps
- Frying flour
- Kamut
- Lager
- Malt
- Maltodextrin
- Malt vinegar
- Malted liquor
- Meat, especially lunch meats
- Miso (unless made with rice koji)
- Modified food starch
- Oats (*see* Appendix and Resources *section for a list of certified gluten-free oats*)
- Pasta
- Rye
- Seitan ("wheat meat")
- Semolina pasta
- Snack foods with seasonings
- Soup thickeners
- Soups with vegetable protein
- Soy sauce
- Soy milk if sweetened with malt
- Spelt
- Spice and seasoning mixes (e.g. for packaged foods)
- Tea and coffee alternatives
- Triticale
- Udon noodles
- Vegetable starch
- Wheat
- Wheat bran
- Wheat flour
- Wheat germ
- Wheat starch
- Worcestershire sauce

As noted previously, recent research has shown that some brands of rice and some products containing corn have been contaminated by wheat and/or gluten-containing grains. Currently, some brands of rice are genetically-modified. Considering the increased incidence of celiac disease, I recommend checking the source of your rice products and/or buying organic products whenever possible. Certified organic foods are grown without genetically-modified ingredients.

Foods Containing Salicylates and Amines

Salicylates are a family of plant chemicals found naturally in many fruits, vegetables, nuts, herbs and spices, jams, honey, yeast extracts, tea and coffee, juices, beer and wines. They are also present in flavorings (e.g. peppermint), perfumes, scented toiletries, eucalyptus oils, and some medications.

Amines result from the breakdown of amino acids. Large amounts are present in cheese, chocolate, wines, beer, yeast extracts and fish products. They are also found in certain fruits and vegetables such as bananas, avocados, tomatoes and broadbeans.

Many people are sensitive to foods that contain salicylates and amines. As with other food allergy or sensitivity, salicylates and amines can cause digestive problems and neurologic complaints such as headaches, muscle aches, fatigue, mood issues, etc.

Here is a list of foods that may contain salicylates and amines:

SA = both salicylates and amines present

- Alfalfa
- Almonds (SA)
- Almond extract/ flavoring
- Allspice
- Anise
- Apples (including apple juice, cider and cider vinegar); Granny Smith particularly high
- Apricots
- Artichoke
- Asparagus
- Aspirin
- Avocado (SA)
- BHA/BHT
- Basil
- Bay leaf

- Beer (SA)
- Beetroot
- Bell peppers (capsicum)
- Berries (see on this list)
- Blackberries
- Blueberries
- Boysenberries
- Brandy (SA)
- Brazil nuts (SA)
- Broadbean (SA)
- Broccoli (SA)
- Carrot
- Cashews, roasted (SA)
- Catsup
- Cauliflower (SA)
- Cayenne
- Cherries

- Chili peppers
- Chinese vegetables
- Chicory
- Chocolate (SA)
- Cinnamon
- Coconut and coconut products (SA)
- Coffee (decaf contains less)
- Cola (SA)
- Corn (cornmeal, sweet corn, polenta, chips, Cornflakes®, etc.)
- Cloves
- Cranberry
- Cucumbers (including pickles)
- Cumin

- Currants
- Curry
- Dates (SA)
- Date sugar (SA)
- Dill
- Eggplant (SA)
- Endive
- Excedrin®
- Figs (SA)
- Fig syrup (SA)
- Five spice
- Fruit spread (made from salicylate/amine fruits)
- Garam masala
- Gherkin (SA)
- Gooseberries
- Grapefruit (SA)
- Grapes (including dried raisins, wine and wine vinegar: *White vinegar is ok.* (SA)
- Gravies (SA)
- Green olives
- Green peppers
- Guava
- Hazelnuts (SA)
- Honey
- Ketchup
- Kiwi (SA)
- Jam/jelly (made from salicylate/amine fruits)
- Lettuce (except iceberg)
- Lemon (SA)
- Licorice (SA)

- Lime
- Loganberry
- Macadamia nuts (SA)
- Mandarin oranges (SA)
- Mint
- Muesli (SA)
- Mulberry
- Mushrooms (SA)
- Mustard
- Nectarines
- Nitrates/Nitrites
- Olives and olive oil (SA)
- Onion
- Oranges (and orange juice) (SA)
- Oregano
- Paprika
- Parsnip
- Passionfruit (SA)
- Pastes (fish, meat, tomato) (SA)
- Peaches
- Peanuts (SA)
- Pecans (SA)
- Pepper (black/white/red)
- Peppermint
- Pickles
- Pineapple (SA)
- Pine nuts (SA)
- Pimento
- Pistachio (SA)
- Plums (SA)
- Port (SA)

- Potato with skin (new or red; white potatoes ok)
- Prepared marinades and sauces (made from salicylate or amine foods) (SA)
- Prune (SA)
- Pumpkin
- Radish
- Raisins (SA)
- Raspberry (SA)
- Red dye (#40)
- Red peppers
- Rhubarb
- Rosemary
- Rum (SA)
- Sage
- Salami (SA)
- Sausage (SA)
- Sauerkraut
- Seasoned meats and chicken (SA)
- Sesame seeds (also sesame oil and tahini) (SA)
- Sherry (SA)
- Snow peas/sprouts
- Soft drinks (SA)
- Spearmint
- Spinach (SA)
- Sports drinks
- Stock cubes (SA)
- Strawberries
- Sunflower seeds (SA)
- Sweet potato

- Tandoori-style cuisine (made from salicylate or amine foods) (SA)
- Tangerine/tangelo (SA)
- Tarragon
- Tea, black (or herbal tea made from fruits high in salicylates/ amines)
- Thyme
- Tomatoes (and tomato products and tomato juice) (SA)
- Turmeric
- Turnip
- Vanilla extract or flavoring
- Vinegar (cider, red and white wine) (SA)
- Walnuts (also walnut oil) (SA)
- Water chestnuts
- Watercress
- Watermelon
- Wine/cordial (SA)
- Wintergreen
- Worchestershire sauce
- Yeast extracts (SA)
- Yellow dyes (#5 and #6)
- Zucchini

I include this list for those with multiple sensitivities because many of the recipes include nuts, fruits, vegetables, coconut and chocolate. If you have numerous sensitivities, when possible, choose certified organic foods (grown without pesticides and genetically-modified ingredients).

REFERENCES:

1. *Salicylates, Amines and MSG* by Anne Swain, Robert Loblay, Velencia Soutter. Department of Clinical Immunology, Royal Prince Alfred Hospital, Australia, 1991.
2. *Food Chemical Sensitivity: Hyperactive Behavior and Food Additives.* http://www.feingold.org/Research/adhd.html

Foods Containing Tree Nuts

Generally, tree nuts refer to almonds, Brazil nuts, cashews, hazelnuts (filberts), macadamia nuts, pecans, pine nuts (pignolias), pistachios and walnuts. Many of these nuts are in different food families so having an allergic reaction and/or sensitivity to one of the nuts, does not guarantee a sensitivity to all of them. For instance, people sensitive to peanuts may not be sensitive to other nuts. Peanuts are more closely related to soy than to almonds. I do not recommend eating peanuts because they contain aflatoxins. Those without nut sensitivities may enjoy tree nuts instead of peanuts.

Considering the increased incidence of nut allergies (many of which cause analphylaxis reactions), it is often advised that people avoid eating tree nuts. This is especially important for those whose family members have nut allergies or negative reactions to eating nuts. There are some nuts that are not considered tree nuts, despite the "nut" in their names. These include chestnuts, coconut and nutmeg.

For someone who tolerates seeds, seed butters are common replacements for nut butters in recipes (e.g. pumpkin, sunflower, or hemp).

Here is a list of foods that may contain tree nuts:

- Almond paste
- Amaretto
- Asian foods
- Baked goods
- Battered foods
- Brazil nuts
- Breakfast cereals
- Candy bars and desserts
- Cashews
- Chestnuts (technically not considered tree nuts)
- Chili
- Chinese food
- Cookies
- Egg rolls
- Frangelico liqueur
- Hazelnuts (filberts)
- Hickory nuts
- Ice cream
- Macadamia nuts
- Margarine
- Marzipan
- Milk-based formula
- Milkshakes
- Nougat
- Nut butters
- Nut meal
- Nut oil
- Nut paste
- Pastry
- Pecans
- Pesto
- Pine nuts (pignolias)
- Pistachios
- Pralines
- Satay
- Soups
- Thai food
- Vegetable fat
- Vegetable oil
- Walnuts
- Worcestershire sauce

Foods Containing Wheat

Currently some varieties of wheat and rice are also genetically-modified. Considering the increased incidence of celiac disease, I recommend checking the source of your wheat and rice products and/or buying organic whenever possible. Certified organic foods are grown without genetically-modified ingredients.

For those who are not sensitive to wheat, choosing whole wheat products is advised. Labels for more nutrient-dense wheat products will include "whole wheat" in the ingredient list. These foods will provide more protein, fiber and other nutrients.

As mentioned on page 60, blood tests are available to determine if you or a family member are sensitive to gluten and/or have celiac disease. In addition, "gene tests" can also be used to exclude celiac disease, especially if blood test results are inconclusive. *I mention it again here since wheat products inherently contain gluten.* The symptoms of this disease can be "silent" in that they may be easily attributable to other conditions such as stress. Celiac is commonly overlooked, although the rates of incidence are on the rise perhaps due to current research and the damaging effects celiac may cause.

If you have tested negative for wheat intolerance and allergy (IgG and IgE, respectively), celiac disease and gluten intolerance, but continue to notice symptoms, you may be sensitive to a substance in wheat called wheat germ agglutinin (WGA). This substance is found in high concentrations in both sprouted wheat and whole wheat and can have a variety of adverse effects on the body. To read more about this topic, please see the articles by Sayer Ji noted in the *Bibliography* on pages 319-320. Dr. Gabriel Cousens has also written about research on lectins (sugar-binding proteins) in his book, *Conscious Eating*, and other publications.

Here is a list of foods that may contain wheat:

- All-purpose flour
- Baked goods
- Baking powder
- Battered foods
- Bran
- Bread crumbs
- Breaded foods
- Bulgur
- Burgers
- Candy
- Cereal binders
- Cereal extract
- Cereal fillers
- Cereal protein
- Cereal starch
- Cereal, hot and cold
- Corn bread
- Couscous
- Crackers
- Croquettes
- Dextrin
- Durum
- Farina
- Gluten
- Graham crackers
- Grain coffee substitute
- Granola
- Gravy
- Hydrolyzed plant protein
- Hydrolyzed vegetable protein
- Icing
- Instant cocoa
- Kamut
- Lunch meats
- Maltodextrin
- Matzo
- Meatballs
- Meatloaf
- Modified food starch
- Ovaltine®
- Pancakes
- Pasta
- Pie crusts
- Postum
- Processed meats
- Salad dressings
- Sauces
- Sausages
- Seasonings
- Semolina
- Soups
- Soy sauce
- Spelt
- Stabilizers
- Stuffing
- Surimi
- Tamari (wheat-free brands are ok)
- Tempura
- Triticale flour
- Whole wheat flour (pastry or regular)

CHAPTER 11

Superfoods

for Use in Sweet Treats

*Behave so the aroma of your actions may enhance
the general sweetness of the atmosphere.*

-Henry David Thoreau

There are many ways to improve your health, not the least of which is removing sugar from your diet. Foods with additional nutritional value can easily be incorporated into our diets. Consuming fiber and leafy greens (containing minerals) can help reverse diabetes and improve a variety of health conditions. Adding these foods to snacks or treats gives these items even more "staying power."

Here is a list of some delicious superfoods to add to your sweet treats. Many of these items are used in the recipes in this book.

❃ **Acai** (AAH SIGH EEE) is a berry that is high in antioxidants. It can be found in powdered or frozen forms. The frozen form is available in two varieties: with added sugar or raw without added sugar. Acai also provides some omega fats and tastes great when added to smoothies or eaten "as is" like a fruit popsicle. Look for the frozen packets without sweetener added. This gives a whole new meaning to those Technicolor™ fruit stick pops. (*Keep in mind that the pulp often contains guarana, a form of caffeine.*)

❃ **Blue-green algae** is also sometimes referred to as cyanobacteria. It is high in antioxidants and helps minimize free radicals in our bodies. It usually comes in a powdered form and can be used similarly to spirulina powder. *Individuals with extreme food* *sensitivities or the genetic condition phenylketonuria (PKU) may have allergic reactions to algae that contains phenylalanine. For this reason, it is best to select brands of blue-green algae that are independently tested and/or that have assays proving their purity. See the* Appendix and Resources *section on page 312 for the algae sources I recommend.*

❈ **CACAO** is also known as raw chocolate. It comes in many forms: powder, cacao butter (which is creamy), beans (the fruit) or in bits, like a chocolate chip. Raw cacao is high in magnesium and also contains iron. It is delicious blended in smoothies, added to baked goods, mixed with yacon syrup or eaten plain (start with a little as it can taste bitter). Studies have shown that people who eat 50 grams of chocolate (containing at least 70% cacao) per week have lower risks of developing a stroke and dying from a stroke. Because cacao contains caffeine, people who are sensitive should consume cacao in moderation. Recent research indicates concern with the introduction of more cacao into our food supply. *Some people experience problems after consuming cacao: addictive and digestive issues, sleep disturbances, and mood swings. If you choose to consume chocolate, I advocate eating cacao in moderation. Important: Do not feed cacao to your pet. Even one to two ounces of dark chocolate or cacao can be toxic to their systems.*

❈ **CAMU CAMU BERRY** is a berry from the Amazon that is very high in vitamin C. It also contains levels of B vitamins, antioxidants, iron, potassium and bioflavinoids. For an extra boost, add camu camu berry to smoothies and bars.

❈ **CHIA SEEDS** are high in fiber, which helps slow the body's process of converting carbohydrates into sugar. This translates into less blood sugar fluctuation and a reduction in sweet cravings. Chia seeds are rich in omega 3 fatty acids, calcium, boron and antioxidants. They are members of the mint family.

❈ **COCONUT OIL** is a saturated fat. However, it is free of cholesterol, trans-fatty acids and hydrogenated fat. *See Chapter 7 on page 39 for more about coconut oil.*

❈ **E3 LIVE**™ is a form of blue-green algae (specifically, Aphanizomenon flos-aquae or AFA for short) containing

64 easily-absorbed vitamins, minerals and enzymes. Regular ingestion of E3 Live™ has been shown to help balance blood sugar abnormalities. *See the note above for more about blue-green algae.*

✳ **Fruits Of The Earth**™ contains a blend of organically grown high antioxidant fruits, alkalizing vegetables, probiotics, and chromium, which supports healthy blood sugar balance. This can be added to smoothies, truffles, toppings and more. Some of the fruits include blueberry, acai, goji berries and pomegranate.

✳ **Goji berries** are high in amino acids, trace minerals, iron and B vitamins, and they contain all eight essential amino acids (the ones our body can't make). They have been proven to strengthen the immune system. Resembling red raisins, goji berries are part of the nightshade family. Thus, people who react to tomatoes, potatoes or eggplant may also be sensitive to goji berries.

✳ **Greens** include fresh lettuces, kale, Swiss chard from your garden, local farmers, local farmer's market and/or your local grocery store. There are a number of supplemental forms also available to help increase your intake of greens *(see the Appendix and Resources section on pages 312-314).*

✳ **Hemp** is high in digestible protein, vitamin E, iron and omega 3 fatty acids. It can be added to smoothies, eaten plain, sprinkled on a salad, made into hemp milk and, added to muffins and baked goods. Store in a cool, dry place in a dark bottle with little or no exposure to light. Raw hempseeds are also rich, nutty and flavorful and can be eaten in a myriad of ways.

✳ **Incan berries** have been mistakenly referred to as goji berries. Incan berries are high in niacin, beta carotene, vitamin C, bioflavinoids, phosphorus, thiamin and protein. They also help to moderate stress and support the immune system. These berries can be added to cookies, bars, smoothies and more.

✳ **Lucuma powder** (LOO KU MAH) is made from a fruit found in the Peruvian highlands. It has a slightly sweet flavor along with carbohydrates, fiber, calcium, phosphorus, iron and beta carotene. It is a tasty topping and a nice addition to smoothies, raw treats and more.

* **MACA** is an herb that comes from the high altitudes of Peru. It is rich in minerals, essential fatty acids and fiber. It has been shown to increase stamina, increase libido, regulate hormones, and balance mood. It is usually found in a powdered form that can be added to baked goods, smoothies, raw bon bon treats and more.

* **MAQUI BERRY** is new to the market. It is a purple berry indigenous to the Patagonia region of South America and has been enjoyed by the Mapuche Indian people for hundreds of years. This berry contains anythocyanins and is high in antioxidants and polyphenols, both helpful in combating free radicals. Maqui berries also contain vitamin C, calcium, iron and potassium. Though this berry appears to have higher antioxidant levels than acai or other berries, you may wish to consume it in moderation until further research is available.

* **MESQUITE POD POWDER** is ground from the bean pods of the mesquite tree. It has a distinct aroma and can be used as a condiment for additional flavor (or subtle sweetening) in a variety of foods including smoothies, raw treats, pies, sauces and soups. The seed contains protein, amino acids, calcium, magnesium, iron, zinc, lysine and potassium.

* **MULBERRIES** are berries with a distinctive taste. They are high in iron, protein and vitamin C. They are delicious on their own, or when mixed with cacao, smoothies or other treats.

* **PURE SYNERGY**® contains organic and wild-crafted algae, phytonutrients, green juices, Asian mushrooms, Chinese herbs and enzymes. It is a green powder that can be added to bon bons, smoothies, sauces and more. *See the note above for more about blue-green algae.*

* **RAW NUTS AND SEEDS** are often available at local health food stores along with other raw, organic and biodynamically grown

foods. Look for a variety of nuts and seeds such as almonds[*], sunflower, pumpkin, Brazil nuts, walnuts, cashews, pine nuts and macadamia nuts. Nuts and seeds are a great way for those without nut/seed sensitivities to consume more raw foods.

✳ **Raw Power!™ Protein Superfood Supplement** comes in four flavors: vanilla, chocolate, plain and green. It contains many of the superfoods on this list and has a rich nutty flavor and texture. Each flavor contains hemp protein, maca, Brazil nut protein, and more. The raw ingredients have not been heated and provide a super way to add more raw, nutrient-dense foods to your diet.

✳ **Spirulina** includes a range of cyanobacteria and blue-green algae. Composed of 65% protein, spirulina contains all eight essential amino acids. It comes in powder form and can be mixed into smoothies, soups or hot cereal. *See the note above for more about blue-green algae.*

✳ **Sun Warrior Protein®** is not just protein powder; it's a raw superfood made from rice protein that can even be enjoyed by those with food sensitivities. Available in several flavors and sweetened with stevia, Sun Warrior® tastes delicious in smoothies and raw treats. Though a raw product, it can also be used in baked goods.

✳ **Vitamineral Green™** contains organic and wild-crafted whole food vitamin and mineral nutrients in a powder blend. This is like taking your daily multivitamin in a highly-absorbable powdered form. It provides these necessary ingredients of amino acids, antioxidants, chlorophyll, fiber, fatty acids, and probiotics (healthy bacteria for your gut). Consuming Vitamineral Green™ is also a way to incorporate many superfoods into your diet. Unlike many commercial vitamins that contain unnecessary binders, fillers and additional ingredients, Vitamineral Green™ is an alkalizing, very potent food. If you have a sensitive system, use this in small quantities.

---

[*] *Recent laws have mandated that almonds be pasteurized. Please check with your health food store to determine if the almonds they carry are still considered raw. To ease digestion of raw nuts and seeds, you may wish to soak and dry your seeds. Please see the information noted on the* Soaking and Sprouting Chart *on page 134.*

CHAPTER 12:

Sweeteners

in the Sugar Aisle

If you look for sweetness
Your search will be endless
You will never be satisfied
But if you seek the true taste
You will find what you are looking for.

-Buddhist Axiom

Grocery stores frequently add new sweeteners to their aisles—a fact that may help spread the sugar epidemic and also encourage obesity. Due to the plethora of choices available today (with more products entering the market at a rapid pace), we consumers must decipher the differences between these well-marketed items. Making educated choices will help change the way our foods are manufactured. When we take the time to support our local farmers and choose natural, wholesome foods, we help make positive changes in our food supply.

Here is a list of current products found in the sweetener aisle. This list includes some alternative sweeteners. *Please see the charts on pages 92-95 for my recommendations (as of this printing).* Many of the items on this list may sound scientific but they still signify sugar.

I also recommend working with a healthcare practitioner to determine the best transitional sweeteners for you as you omit refined sugar from your diet.

✳ **AGAVE SYRUP** (AAH GAV EH) is derived from the sap of the agave cactus plant, a native predominately to Mexico and Central America. There are over 300 species of agave and the one found most often in our current food supply is from the agave tequilana or blue agave. Though frequently compared to honey (due to its color), agave pours easily, does not crystallize, and has a shelf life of up to three years.

The sap is heated to create the syrup we purchase in the store (if it wasn't, it would be tequila!) Agave is sold in dark, amber and light varieties. The darker the color, the lower the glycemic index and the higher the mineral content. Some recent research indicates a level of toxic impurities present in the darker varieties of agave syrup. Many prefer using the lighter varieties for recipes to achieve their desired result of sweetness without a change in taste.

Proven to alter blood sugar, agave can also contribute to candida and a more acidic condition in the body. Some people have reported sensitivity reactions to agave. Although agave has been marketed as a natural sweetener, even raw agave has been heated from its natural state to create the sweet taste.

Some manufacturers note "suitable for diabetics" on the label, however, for diabetics struggling with blood sugar imbalance, I recommend testing agave to see how the body responds. Because agave is fructose, those sensitive to fructose in other forms may also respond negatively to agave syrup. Fructose is metabolized by the body unlike glucose; in high quantities, it is detrimental to our health. Fructose is sweeter than sucrose, so less agave is needed to create a sweetened product. Though most people rarely add less agave (or other alternative sweeteners) to their food (though agave and alternatives are "sweeter" than sugar), those people still benefit from consuming less calories (than sugar) per serving. To keep up with the increasing demand for agave, some manufacturers have been adding corn syrup to their agave to lower costs and accelerate the processing. This can lead to reactions in corn-sensitive individuals, and change how the sweetener is metabolized, sometimes resulting in obesity and complications related to heart disease.

Some of my clients have reacted to agave nectar. Their symptoms include fatigue, lethargy, "phlegmy throat," tooth pain or discomfort, spiked blood sugar (upon finger pricking) and a "buzz" similar to the feeling of having eaten refined sugar.

While pregnant for the first time, with our son, I was diagnosed with gestational diabetes. Over two years later, while pregnant with our daughter, I used 50 grams of agave for my gestational diabetes test. When I tested with the agave (instead of drinking the "usual" solution), my tests came back normal. Although my food cravings and tolerable food choices were different when I was pregnant with my son than when I was pregnant with our daughter, I wondered if ingesting the highly sweetened and chemical- laden prescription of bright green or bright pink liquid (the glucose solution) altered my blood glucose levels.

This is not medical advice, rather, a possible suggestion for other pregnant women to discuss with a midwife or OB-GYN. If you prefer, you may want to consider using 50 grams of a different alternative sweetener for your test (e.g. brown rice syrup, yacon syrup or one from those listed on page 92).

❋ **Amasake** (AMMA SOCK EH) is a traditional Japanese product made by fermenting sweet brown rice into a thick, sweet liquid. It is sold in the refrigerated section of natural foods stores or in aseptic packages on the shelf. Amasake can replace not only sweeteners but also dairy products in natural desserts. (Recommended)

❋ **Barley malt** is a maltose liquid with a molasses consistency. It is made from soaked, sprouted, and cooked barley. Barley malt contains gluten and has a malt-like taste. Some malt products can also contain corn and/or MSG. To prevent spoilage, refrigerate this sweetener after opening.

❋ **Beet sugar** is a form of sugar extracted from the common beet. Sugar produced from beets is almost chemically identical to cane sugar. Beets are hardy and grown in temperate climates making beet sugar easier to produce.

❋ **Brown rice syrup** is made from rice that has been soaked, sprouted and cooked with a cereal enzyme that breaks the starches into maltose. Rice syrup looks similar to barley malt, corn syrup and honey but is less sweet. If you are sensitive to gluten, be sure to choose a gluten-free form of this syrup. (Recommended)

❋ **Brown sugar** is refined white sugar with molasses added to create the brown color.

❋ **Caramel** is heated sugar resulting in the characteristic flavor and color.

❋ **Carob** is used in baking (in the form of chips or powder) and comes from a carob tree, a species of evergreen shrub in the pea family. It is derived from the edible pulp of the pod, then ground plain or roasted before grinding. Carob is caffeine-free and has a nutty, bitter, slightly sweet taste. Carob chips, a common substitute for chocolate, are not gluten-free; they are often sweetened with malted barley. (*Some store-bought carob contain corn and/or soy derivatives.*) To substitute unsweetened carob powder for cocoa powder, replace 1 part cocoa with 2 ½ parts carob powder (by weight). Carob syrups are often derived from a species of carob tree unlike the variety used to make powdered carob. Commercially-produced carob syrups are not readily available in stores so, making a syrup using dried carob is often easier. (Recommended)

❋ **Castor or caster sugar** is a finely granulated sugar used in Britain. It is called "berry sugar" in British Columbia.

❋ **Coconut sugar** is derived from the sugar blossoms of the tropical coconut palm tree. The flowers are sliced open to collect the nectar, which is ground into a fine dark brown crystal after kettle-boiling and heat evaporation. Tropical coconut palms are considered an ecologically beneficial tree crop, helping to restore damaged soils, needing very little water and providing jobs for "sugar tappers". Though these trees are called coconut palms, palm oil is produced by a different palm species. Coconut sugar is unbleached, unfiltered and usually organically processed without preservatives. This sugar is high in B vitamins, zinc, iron, potassium and magnesium. This sugar can be used in any of the recipes *(see Part 2)* as a low-glycemic alternative to maple sugar crystals. Current research indicates that consumption of coconut sugar generates safe blood sugar responses in people with diabetes. Sensitive individuals should note that coconut sugar contains high levels of aspartic and glutamic acid. This sugar is sometimes sold as "arenga sugar." Ensure that labels note "100% pure coconut palm sugar" as sometimes it is sold mixed with refined or malt sugars. If fermented, coconut sugar turns to vinegar. As recommended in regard to other sweeteners, I advise having your pH level tested for your personal metabolic type. Since this product is newer to the market, I also advise you regularly review labels and brands to ensure the most accurate information. Store coconut sugar in a cool, dry place to avoid mold growth. (RECOMMENDED)

❋ **CONFECTIONERS OR POWDERED SUGAR**, commonly found in icing, is white sugar that has been ground and then sifted. It contains cornstarch (added to prevent caking).

❋ **DATE SUGAR** is made from dehydrated dates that are ground into a powder. It is a wholesome sweetener that is easier to use for a topping or smoothie than in baked products. One can also make a date paste by soaking dates and blending them with a little bit of the soaking water to make a desired consistency. *Oats are sometimes added during date sugar processing. Ensure that the date sugar you purchase contains either gluten-free oats or is oat-free.* (RECOMMENDED)

❋ **DEXTRAN** is a polysaccharide containing many glucose molecules. Dextran is also formed by *Lactobacillus brevis*, a bacterium.

❋ **DEXTROSE** is a corn-derived form of glucose and commonly referred to on food labels (rather than glucose). Some other names include D-glucose or grape sugar. Sugaridextrose is another name for blended sugar.

❀ **DIASTASE** refers to a group of enzymes which breakdown starch into maltose.

❀ **DIASTATIC MALT** can be used as a sugar substitute in bread. It breaks down and converts the starch in dough to sugars, which feeds the yeast.

❀ **DRIED OR EVAPORATED CANE JUICE** is often noted on the nutritional labels of other foods. It has been extracted from the sugar cane and dehydrated. Unrefined cane juice can be found in Rapadura®. When noted on a product label, cane juice can refer to varying amounts of processed sugar and may be bleached. *With the exception of Rapadura®, most evaporated cane juice brands retain little or no vitamins or minerals. See page 84 to read more about Rapadura®. Dried cane juice will raise blood sugar.*

❀ **EMERALD FOREST™ XYLITOL*** is derived from birch.

❀ **ENLITEN**® is a stevia-based sweetener manufactured by Corn Products U.S. The part of the plant used without adverse effects (in Japan and South America) is stevioside. Numerous studies have shown that stevioside is safe. This product contains Rebaudioside A (Reb A), a different stevia compound that has not been widely tested.

❀ **ERYTHRITOL*** is a sugar alcohol that results from fermenting corn.

❀ **ETHYL MALTOL** is a flavourant added to some sweet foods.

❀ **FLORIDA CRYSTALS**® is evaporated cane juice sugar with molasses removed. As advertised, it is sun-sweetened and carbon-free though it still remains a form of sugar. This company produces a variety of sweetener-related products.

❀ **FROZEN FRUIT CONCENTRATE** can be used as a liquid sweetener once thawed. Choose brands in the freezer section that contain fruit only, with no added sugar. Some of these concentrates contain corn or derivatives of corn. For instance, ascorbic acid, a common preservative, is often derived from corn. Due to processing and pasteurization, there are less nutrients

---

*   *Corn-sensitive individuals may not tolerate products made with xylitol or erythritol.*

in this frozen form than in fresh fruit. Using these concentrates will affect blood sugar. (RECOMMENDED)

❊ **FRUCTOSE** is sometimes referred to as levulose and is derived from sucrose and often high fructose corn syrup. It is even sweeter in taste than table sugar (sucrose). Fructose is available in granulated or crystallized form, and is also a large component of high fructose corn syrup. Also high in fructose are honey and sugar alcohols (e.g. any sugars ending in "-ol" such as xylitol*, sorbitol, etc.), As a result of the manufacturing process, crystalline fructose may contain heavy metals (such as lead and arsenic), and other potentially harmful chemicals and toxins. *To read more about fructose and its effect on blood sugar, please see pages 41-44.*

❊ **FRUCTOOLIGOSACCHARIDES** (FOS), also sometimes referred to as oligofructose, oligofructan or inulin, are indigestible carbohydrates that occur naturally and have a mildly sweet taste. Commonly extracted from chicory root and Jerusalem artichokes, they have been shown to be suitable for diabetics and those with blood sugar imbalance, not effecting blood sugar levels upon ingestion. FOS is commonly seen in probiotic formulations, providing nourishment for bacteria found in our guts and reducing the pH of the colon. This is used as a sweetener in combination with stevia in the ChicoLin™ product.

❊ **FRUITS** provide the most wholesome sweetener from the whole food perspective. However, fruits may be more difficult to digest and assimilate when combined with other ingredients. Fruits often digest most completely when eaten on their own. Additional nutrients are obtained when eating from a variety of fruits including fiber, which naturally slows down the absorption of sugar into the bloodstream. When combined with oil, fat or greens, fruit can be processed in the body without an intense rise in blood sugar. (RECOMMENDED)

---

* *Corn-sensitive individuals may not tolerate products made with xylitol or erythritol.*

❊ **FRUITSOURCE**® consists of fruit pureés purchased from manufacturers and sold to consumers in certain products. Products made with Fruitsource® may contain a blend of brown rice syrup and concentrated grape juice. Fruitsource® is not for commercial sale. (RECOMMENDED)

❊ **FRUITTRIM**® is a non-GMO and gluten-free sweetener free of MSG and corn. It is made from real fruit juice combined with dextrin. Dextrin is a carbohydrate produced by the breakdown of starch used as an additive for flavor and/or color. This sweetener is only sold in large quantities to manufacturers.

❊ **GLYCERINE OR VEGETABLE GLYCERINE** is derived from palm or coconut oils processed under pressure and high heat. It has a sweet taste and a thick, syrupy consistency. Although sometimes offered as a sweetener, glycerine is most often found in cosmetics.

❊ **GOLDEN SUGAR OR SYRUP** is also referred to as refiners syrup, yellow sugar or treacle. It is a form of inverted sugar syrup. The syrup looks like honey and may contain corn derivatives.

❊ **HONEY,** though a wholesome source, is a higher-glycemic alternative sweetener that is high in fructose. There are different kinds of honey. Check labels as some honey contains corn syrup added during processing. It is worth paying slightly more for certified organic honey to avoid toxic chemicals often added during processing. Honey can contribute to candida and a more acidic condition in the body. The highest quality honey is raw and made locally. (*Meet beekeepers in your area and learn about their practices.*) Raw honey (not heated over 117°F) contains enzymes and when consumed, has been shown to help alleviate certain allergies. Manuka Honey is an unpasteurized honey. *Avoid all honey while pregnant and nursing. Never give honey or raw honey to an infant or child under one year of age because it may cause botulism. Some resources suggest that people who are elderly, immunocompromised or taking statin drugs for cholesterol should limit or avoid honey. Speak with a knowledgeable healthcare practitioner for more information.*

❋ **HYDROGENATED STARCH HYDROSYLATE (HSH)** is a generic term referring to the mixture of several sugar alcohols.

❋ **INVERT SUGAR OR SYRUP** is a combination of glucose and fructose that has been broken down. It has a sweeter taste than sucrose (table sugar). Invert sugar is found naturally in maple syrup and honey, and in homemade jam or jelly. However, when listed on a package, it is generally manufactured through one of two ways. Invert sugar is made by adding an acid to sucrose to further break it down, or by using Invertase, a yeast-derived enzyme.

❋ **JERUSALEM ARTICHOKE SYRUP** is new to the market. This syrup is similar to yacon and molasses but has a milder flavor. Comprised of fructose, Jerusalem artichoke syrup is made from the juiced, dehydrated Jerusalem artichoke. This syrup is harvested sustainably and has a very low glycemic index. *For those sensitive to seeds, Jerusalem artichoke is a tuber from the sunflower species. It may also ferment quickly, making it more difficult to use in larger quantities.* (RECOMMENDED)

❋ **JUST LIKE SUGAR**® contains chicory root, maltodextrin, inulin, calcium, vitamin C and natural orange peel. Both inulin and maltodextrin are sugar, and the vitamin C may be corn-derived.

❋ **KATEMFE PLANT FRUIT** is a West African plant (also called "Sweet Prayer Plant"). Its berries contain a sweet protein called thaumatin. (RECOMMENDED)

❋ **LAKANTO**™ is a sweetener from Japan made from erythritol* and luo han guo fruit (from China). Erythritol* is a sugar alcohol that results from fermenting corn.

❋ **LICORICE ROOT** is an herb often used as a sweetener in teas or herbal blends. The official name for this herb is glycyrrhizin. I include it here for those of you who require "hints of sweet." Due to a concern that licorice root may cause edema and/or hypertension with moderate to high consumption, herbalists and other professionals recommend that consumption not

---

* *Corn-sensitive individuals may not tolerate products made with xylitol or erythritol.*

exceed 200 milligrams (according to the most current research at the time of this publication). *Licorice root is entirely different from licorice sticks. The latter are sold in stores and generally contain corn syrup, gluten flours, sugar and preservatives.* (RECOMMENDED)

❈ **LO HAN KUO OR LO HAN GUO** (LOW HAN KOO OH) is a cultivated fruit from China that has a black licorice flavor and is 300 times sweeter than sugar. It is often referred to as the longevity fruit in China, and has little to no calories. It contains no sugar and has a naturally sweet taste. Similar to stevia, this fruit cannot be broken down through human digestion, therefore causing no rise in blood sugar levels. This fruit is in the cucumber, melon, squash and gourd family. (RECOMMENDED)

❈ **LO HAN SWEET**™ is a sweetener sold through Jarrow Formulas® which combines lo han kuo and xylitol*. The xylitol* in this product is sourced from corn.

❈ **LUCUMA POWDER** (LOO KU MAH) is made from a fruit found in the Peruvian highlands. It has a slightly sweet flavor along with carbohydrates and fiber. It also provides calcium, phosphorus, iron and beta carotene. Lucuma powder is a nice addition to smoothies and raw treats, as a topping and more. (RECOMMENDED)

❈ **MALTISORB**® is hydrogenated maltitol.

❈ **MALTISWEET**® is a corn-derived maltitol product offered through Corn Products U.S. This company also offers a large range of other polyol sweeteners. Some other product names include Hystar®, Stabilite®, Sorbogem®, Sorbo®, Erysta®, Xylogem™, and Glystar®. In addition, Corn Products U.S. offers other corn-derived sweeteners such as Cerelose® Dextrose, Cerelose® Anhydrous Dextrose, Unidex® and Royal T® Dextrose, Globe® and Amidex™ Maltodextrins and Corn Syrup Solids, Invertose® High Fructose Corn Syrup, Enliten®, SweetDex™, and Polidex® MD/MDA.

---

* *Corn-sensitive individuals may not tolerate products made with xylitol or erythritol.*

❋ **Maltodextrin** is a food additive commonly found in candy and soda. It is a starch usually derived from either wheat or corn.

❋ **Maltose** is malt sugar, derived from two glucose units.

❋ **Maple syrup/maple sugar crystals** are harvested from maple trees. The sap from the trees is boiled to produce different forms of maple sugar. There are three grades of syrup available, (determined by the processing temperature and length of time cooked): A, B or C. Grade A is best for pancakes and waffles. Grade B has a better flavor for baking, is less expensive and has a higher mineral content. Grade C syrup is for commercial use only. Purchase organic products only because non-organic brands may contain formaldehyde, chemical agents and mold inhibitors. Only pure maple syrup is guaranteed to be free of corn syrup and/or corn derivatives. Maple sugar crystals are less refined than maple syrup. Refrigerate after opening. *This sweetener often raises blood sugar in sugar-sensitive people and those with diabetes.* (Recommended)

❋ **Molasses** is a by-product of the sugar refining process. Sweet molasses is useful as an alternative sweetener to refined cane sugar. Both blackstrap molasses and sweet molasses are rich sources of iron, calcium, potassium, trace minerals and B vitamins. Those nutrients that are unharmed by heating are 30 times more concentrated in molasses than in the original cane juice. If not organic, molasses may contain high amounts of pesticides and sulfur dioxide, an allergen for some people. If you are corn-sensitive, check the molasses you are using to ensure it doesn't contain corn derivatives. Refrigerate after opening or store in a cool, dry location. (Recommended)

❋ **Muscovado sugar** or **Barbados sugar** has a dark brown color and a sticky consistency, both qualities resulting from its naturally high molasses content. It is minimally refined sugar with coarse, rough crystals derived directly from sugarcane juice. Though heated and dried, muscovado sugar retains nutrients like potassium, magnesium, calcium and iron, and it is similar to Rapadura®, an unrefined sweetener. Since this sugar has a high moisture content, it can sometimes be difficult to use with recipes that require baking.

❋ **NATURE SWEET**® by Steel's Gourmet™ contains maltitol, made from corn.

❋ **ORGANIC ZERO**™ is organic erythritol*, a sugar alcohol produced by fermenting cane sugar.

❋ **PANOCHA** refers to a kind of cane sugar in the Philippines.

❋ **POLYDEXTROSE** is formed mainly from dextrose and is classified as a soluble fiber food ingredient.

❋ **POLYOLS** is another name for sugar alcohols. For more information, please see page 87 under "sugar alcohols."

❋ **PUREVIA**™ is stevia (the Reb A variety) plus erythritol* and isomaltulose. This product is being used by PepsiCo, Inc. in their SoBe® Lifewater energy drinks. The variety of stevia used in PureVia™ is processed in China, and may not be as pure as the stevia processed in South America. This is a stevia-based sweetener which may contain other sweetener ingredients.

❋ **RAFFINOSE** is an oigosaccharide found in many vegetables and whole grains. It is a combination of galactose, fructose and glucose. Humans do not have the enzyme needed to breakdown the raffinose family, commonly resulting in flatulence.

❋ **RAPADURA**® (RAH PAH DURA) is unrefined sugar from organically-grown sugar cane produced through fair trade programs in Columbia and Brazil. Rapadura® manufacturing evaporates the water from the organic sugar cane juice, resulting in dried sugar cane crystals. This sugar is unbleached and unrefined, which helps retain some essential vitamins and minerals. Unlike most sugars, Rapadura® is not separated from the molasses during processing. Though not a "health" food, this sugar is hand-processed, and has a crystallized texture and

---

* *Corn-sensitive individuals may not tolerate products made with xylitol or erythritol.*

the color and flavor of caramel. Though unrefined, this is sugar and will affect blood sugar. (RECOMMENDED)

❋ RAW SUGAR, though less refined than white sugar, has still been heated. In some cases, the brown color of raw sugar results from the addition of molasses after processing. Raw sugar has all the properties of refined white sugar.

❋ SLIM & SWEET™ also referred to as SlimSweet™, contains lo han kuo and levulose (another name for fructose).

❋ SMART SWEET® xylitol* granules are non-GMO and derived from birch. *This brand name also manufactures sweeteners containing erythritol and other non-recommended ingredients. Be sure to ask for the xylitol* sweetener only.*

❋ SOOOO SWEET!® is a stevia product made with the Rebiana A part of the plant.

❋ SORGHUM (SORE GUM) is a grass-like plant that is processed into a light brown syrup or grain flour. It is also used in some alcoholic beverages and for biofuel. It has a molasses-like taste. Sorghum products may be contaminated by corn.

❋ STEVIA (STEE VEE UH) is a plant from the daisy family that grows naturally in South America. The plant contains stevioside, which, in powdered extract form, is estimated to be 300 times as sweet as table sugar. In leaf form, stevia is 15 to 30 times sweeter than sugar. It has no calories, is suitable for diabetics, helps to balance the pancreas, fights cavities, is safe for children, heat-stable (e.g. acceptable for baking), and has been researched and used in many countries around the world. Stevia is an antifungal, anti-inflammatory and antibiotic agent. It is available as a white or green powder and in liquid form. It can also combine with other natural sugars such as honey, maple sugar and molasses.

Stevia liquid is great in teas, shakes, puddings and drinks. The green, less processed variety, is slightly more bitter than the white variety. White or clear stevia is often refined and can lead

---

* *Corn-sensitive individuals may not tolerate products made with xylitol or erythritol.*

to sugar imbalance. I recommend brown or green stevia liquids or powders. Stevia liquid is also available in different flavors (*see the* Appendix and Resources *section on page 296 for more information*).

Some larger manufacturers such as Cargill, The Coca-Cola Company, and PepsiCo, are now researching the use of stevia (labeling it rebiana) and sourcing the plant from China rather than South America. Some of these stevia-based sweeteners are made with Rebiana A, a different component of the stevia plant. This part of the plant has not been widely researched and I recommend knowing more about the source before choosing to incorporate it into your diet. Some stevia manufacturers may use alcohols, enzymes or chemicals during processing, which can change the herb's makeup and reduce its natural benefits.

Using stevia in baked products requires experimentation because very little is needed to achieve the sweet taste. The ratios of dry and wet ingredients also need to be altered in order to achieve the desired texture, mouth feel and overall delicious result.

Stevia is now considered a food additive and has been determined (by the World Health Organization) to be safe for consumption as a sweetener to use (up to 4 mg of stevia per kg of body weight, per day). Avoid the combined sweeteners that contain stevia (e.g. PureVia™, Stevia in the Raw™ and Truvia™, as noted on pages 74-90). Dr. Gabriel Cousens has researched stevia in the reversal of diabetes. His most recent book is called *There is a Cure for Diabetes*. (RECOMMENDED)

❅ STEVIA BY XYMOGEN® contains maltodextrin and the Rebiana A stevia from Columbia. It is a non-GMO, organic product.

❅ STEVIA IN THE RAW™ is stevia sold in packets through Sweet N' Low® brands. The sourcing of this stevia may not be pure and may contain other ingredients.

❅ SUCANAT™ (SOO KA NOT) stands for "sugar cane natural." It is organically grown dried sugar cane juice with molasses added. It is processed through dehydration (as opposed to evaporation for Rapadura®). It has a lower sucrose content than traditional and refined table sugar and is grainy rather than crystalline in texture. If the Sucanat™ you purchase has a darker color (similar to Rapadura®), it is likely less refined. Another cane juice processed like Sucanat™ is Alter Eco™.

❇ **Sugar alcohols** include a variety of sweeteners. Some of these include erythritol*, isomalt, lactitol, mannitol, maltitol, maltol, sorbitol and xylitol*. Sugar alcohols occur naturally in low amounts in some raw fruits and vegetables. When people eat processed foods containing processed sugar alcohols, they often ingest more sugar alcohols than they would if they ate a piece of fruit, which contains naturally-occuring sugar alcohols. Products made with sugar alcohols will generally have fewer calories than foods sweetened with sugar. However, most of these sweeteners have been shown to alter blood sugar and cause digestive side effects. Because the majority of sugar alcohols are derived from genetically-modified corn, they pose a health risk. Consuming organic or birch-derived xylitol* in small amounts (such as ¼ tsp to 1 tsp) has been shown to decrease and/or prevent tooth decay.

❇ **Sugar in the Raw**® is granulated (and refined) turbinado sugar and is sold through Sweet N' Low® brands.

❇ **SugarNot**™ contains lo han kuo fruit and corn-derived fructose.

❇ **Sun Crystals**® contain raw cane sugar and stevia.

❇ **Sweet & Slender**® contains a combination of fructose and lo han guo.

❇ **Sweeten Me**® contains erythritol* (from non-GMO corn), inulin, FOS blend, fructose, citric extract and flavor. It is a GMO-free product.

❇ **SweetLIFE**™ is now referred to as Slim & Sweet™ or SlimSweet™. It contains lo han kuo and levulose (fructose).

❇ **Sweet Perfection**™ contains FOS or oligofructose.

---

* *Corn-sensitive individuals may not tolerate products made with xylitol or erythritol.*

❋ **Sweet Serum**™ contains yacon, stevia, and Xagave™ (a raw agave with a patented process).

❋ **Sweet Simplicity**® contains erythritol* and fructose (levulose).

❋ **Tapioca Syrup** is known by other names such as cassava, yucca, manioc or mandioc. These roots are found in tropical climates of South America. The syrup is converted from the raw root with the use of natural enzymes. Tapioca syrup has a neutral taste and can replace liquid sweeteners in recipes with relative ease. (Recommended)

❋ **TheraSweet**™ is xylitol* plus tagatose.

❋ **The Ultimate Sweetener**® contains xylitol*, a sugar alcohol. Its source is from birch rather than corn. This product is processed in Finland, where pesticides are not used.

❋ **Trehalose** has a sweet and mild flavor and is often used in a variety of processed foods. It is not generally used to replace sucrose in recipes.

❋ **Truvia**™, found in Vitaminwater Zero® and Recharge® (and other drink products) is a combination of rebiana (from the leaf of the stevia plant) and erythritol*. It may also contain other sweetener ingredients. The Coca-Cola and Cargill companies are working to research and produce rebiana.

❋ **Turbinado** sugar is made from the extracted sugar cane juice that is evaporated (with heat). The resulting brown crystals are spun in a turbine to remove excess water, thus the name. Turbinado is often used for either white or brown sugar in recipes. This is still sugar and is sometimes referred to as Demerara.

❋ **Xlear Inc**® or **XyloSweet**® contains xylitol* only. The xylitol* in this sweetener is sourced from corn.

❋ **Xylitol*** (Z-EYE LEE TALL) is also called wood sugar or birch sugar, and is a sugar alcohol that is used as a sugar substitute. It can be extracted from birch, raspberries, plums, and corn and is primarily produced in China.

*   *Corn-sensitive individuals may not tolerate products made with xylitol or erythritol.*

Xylitol*, gram for gram, is roughly as sweet as sucrose, but contains 40% less food energy than sucrose. Absorbed more slowly than sugar, it doesn't contribute to high blood sugar levels or the resulting hyperglycemia caused by insufficient insulin response. As a sugar alcohol, xylitol* is only partially absorbed by the body, lessening its effect on blood sugar levels. However, xylitol* is high in fructose and sensitive individuals will benefit from consuming it in moderation.

Like other sugar alcohols, xylitol* may cause gas, bloating and diarrhea in amounts greater than four grams (e.g. four pieces of gum). People with irritable bowel syndrome may have difficulty digesting xylitol*. Preliminary research has shown xylitol* to be effective in preventing tooth decay, ear and upper respiratory infections, and oral candida (yeast). It has also been shown to help cellular response to Vitamin D3, which, in certain dosages, can help to prevent and reverse osteopenia and osteoporosis.

In the U.S., xylitol* is approved as a food additive (in unlimited quantity) for foods with special dietary purposes. To avoid the possibility of buying a product containing genetically-modified corn, choose products labeled "made from birch sugar." I recommend you enjoy this sweetener in small amounts, e.g. in a piece of gum, or sprinkled on top of sliced fruit. *A small amount of xylitol* (e.g. one or two pieces of gum) can be toxic if consumed by your pet.* (RECOMMENDED)

❋ YACON SYRUP (Yaah CONE) is from the yacon plant native to South America. It is a low-glycemic syrup-like sweetener (from the root of the plant) which is also high in antioxidants and fructooligosaccharides (FOS), or beneficial bacteria found in our digestive system. With current dietary ingestion, many people are low in these beneficial bacteria. FOS can help us absorb vitamins and minerals with more ease. Some yacon syrups are heat-treated. If you are looking for a raw sweetener, ask the manufacturer if they have a variety that has not been heated above 118°F. (RECOMMENDED)

---

* *Corn-sensitive individuals may not tolerate products made with xylitol or erythritol.*

❋ **Z Sweet**® is made from erythritol* and natural fruit sweeteners.

❋ **Zerose**™ is made from erythritol* and introduced by Cargill, Incorporated.

Recommended Steps Toward Replacing Sugar with Alternative Sweeteners

People often ask me to rank the sweeteners or make a step-by-step process for eliminating, reducing and/or omitting sugar from one's diet. Though my recommendations are always tailored to the individual, I offer the following to help you adjust your relationship with sugar.

1. Immediately remove any artificial sweeteners (*as noted in the list on page 13*) from your diet. These sweeteners are neurotoxins (toxic to the brain) and not healthy for anyone's consumption. For example, you could decrease the amount of soda with a goal of omitting it entirely. (*See page 128 for a recipe for a soda substitute.*) A study performed at Harvard School of Public Health concluded that individuals consuming more than one sweetened beverage per day substantially increased their risk of gaining weight and developing diabetes.

2. Remove refined, processed sugar from your diet. See the chart on pages 94-95 as a guide.

3. Consider purchasing a glucose monitor at your local drugstore. Monitors currently cost approximately $25. (Glucose strips are an additional fee.) During this phase of shifting from traditional sugars to alternative sweeteners, you can test your blood sugar to learn how your body personally responds to the different alternatives. If you are interested, I can provide a chart to help you monitor your findings.

4. Lastly, begin choosing from the list of alternative sweeteners on page 92. Please note that many of the alternatives, though not artificial, have varying glycemic indexes, are manufactured, may cause side effects in sensitive people, encourage weight gain and

---

*   *Corn-sensitive individuals may not tolerate products made with xylitol or erythritol.*

alter both insulin sensitivity and the alkaline/acidic balance in your body.

These alternatives are not created equal. After you remove artificial and refined sweeteners from your diet, I advise that you consume alternative sweeteners in moderation. For example, the most recent publicity related to agave nectar highlights the importance of listening to your own intuition when experimenting with alternative sweeteners. Although having been marketed as a low glycemic sweetener, agave still requires personal consideration. Using this book as a resource while upgrading your current sweetener choices can include incorporating agave in moderation.

Please remember that according to the USDA (as of 2003), most people consumed an average of almost 13 teaspoons of refined sugar per day (more than ¼ of a cup). Taking any of these steps is a vast improvement!

If you would like help navigating through alternatives best suited for your needs, please contact me for a private counseling session.

Don't ask what the world needs.
Ask what makes you come alive, and go do that.
Because what the world needs is people who have come alive.
-Howard Thurman

Guide to Sweeteners*

Recommended Sweeteners

❋ Amasake

❋ Brown rice syrup

❋ Carob or carob syrup

❋ Coconut palm sugar (organic without added sugars)

❋ Date sugar

❋ Frozen fruit concentrate (no added sugars)

❋ Fruit, fresh

❋ Fruitsource® (available only as ingredient in other products)

❋ Jerusalem artichoke syrup

❋ Katemfe plant fruit

❋ Licorice root (not sticks)

❋ Lo han kuo

❋ Lucuma powder

❋ Organic maple syrup or maple sugar crystals (containing no corn syrup or formaldehyde)

❋ Molasses

❋ Rapadura®

❋ Stevia**

❋ Tapioca syrup

❋ Xylitol *** (derived from birch only and GMO-free)

❋ Yacon syrup

---

*   *For more details, please see descriptions on pages 74-90.*
** *Stevia is difficult to use with consistent results in vegan and gluten-free baking. I recommend using it in the recipes where it is noted. Stevia is safe for diabetics and people with candida. Not all brands of stevia are the same. See the Appendix and Resource section on page 296 for quality stevia sources.*
*** *Corn-sensitive individuals may not tolerate products made with xylitol or erythritol.*

*Transitional Sweeteners**

❋ Agave syrup or nectar (organic and blue agave)

❋ Barley malt/malt syrup (contains gluten)

❋ ChicoLin™

❋ Dehydrated organic sugar cane juice

❋ Dried organic cane juice

❋ Erythritol** if organic and GMO-free (usually corn-derived)

❋ Evaporated organic cane juice (another name for dehydrated cane juice)

❋ Florida Crystals®

❋ Honey (local, organic, raw, enzyme-rich)

❋ Lakanto®**

❋ Sorghum or sorghum syrup

❋ Sucanat®

Transitional times will vary between individuals. I recommend skipping this intermediary step (if possible) and experimenting with the recommended sweeteners. Please note these sweeteners will effect blood sugar in variable amounts.

---

*   *Either omit these sweeteners or use occasionally in small amounts (one tablespoon or less). Transitional times will vary between individuals. I suggest that people avoid transitional sweeteners altogether (if possible) and experiment with recommended sweeteners instead. Please note that these transitional sweeteners will effect blood sugar in variable amounts. See the descriptions on pages 74-90 for more details.*

** *Corn-sensitive individuals may not tolerate products made with xylitol or erythritol.*

Sweeteners to Avoid

- Acesulfame potassium
- Acesulfame K
- Ace-K
- Aclame™
- Alitame
- Altern™
- AminoSweet®
- Aspartame
- Aspartic acid
- Barbados sugar
- Beet sugar
- Brown sugar
- Buttered syrup
- Cane juice crystals (unless Rapadura®)
- Cane sugar
- Canderel®
- Caramel
- Castor sugar
- Confectioners sugar
- Corn sugar
- Corn syrup
- Corn syrup solids
- Crystalline dextrose
- Crystalline fructose
- Cyclamate
- Demerara
- Dextran
- Dextrose
- Diastatic malt
- Diastase
- Enliten®
- Equal®
- Ethyl maltol
- Fructose
- Glucose
- Glucose solids
- Glucose syrup
- Glycerine or vegetable glycerine
- Golden sugar
- Golden syrup
- High fructose corn syrup (HFCS)
- Hydrogenated starch hydrolysates
- Hydrolysed starch
- Invert sugar
- Invert syrup
- Isomalt
- Just Like Sugar®
- Lactitol (dairy-derived sugar alcohol)
- Lactose (milk sugar)
- Levulose (fructose)
- Lo Han Sweet™
- Maltitol
- Maltisorb™
- Maltisweet™
- Maltodextrin
- Maltol
- Maltose
- Mannitol
- Muscovado sugar
- Naturlose™
- Neotame
- Novasweet™
- Nutrasweet®
- Nutrasweet 2000®
- Organic Zero™
- P-4000
- Panocha
- Phenylalanine
- Polydextrose
- Powdered sugar
- PureVia™
- Raffinose
- Raw sugar
- Refiners syrup
- Saccharin
- Shugr™
- Slim & Sweet™ or SlimSweet™
- Soooo Sweet!®
- Sorbitol
- Spoonful®
- Splenda®
- Stevia in the Raw™
- Sucralose
- Sucrose
- Sugar
- Sugaridextrose
- Sugar in the Raw®
- SugarTwin®
- Sun Crystals®
- Sunett®
- Sweet & Safe®
- Sweet & Slender®
- Sweetener 2000®

- Sweet Me®
- SweetLIFE®
- Sweet One®
- Sweet Perfection®
- Sweet N' Low®
- Sweet Simplicity®
- Swiss Sweet®

- Tagatose
- Talin™
- TheraSweet™
- Treacle
- Trehalose
- Truvia™
- Turbinado sugar

- Xlear Inc® or XyloSweet®
- Yellow sugar
- Z Sweet®
- Zerose™

CHAPTER 13:

Replacing

Sugar with Alternative Sweeteners*

The intellect says: "The six directions are limits: there is no way out."
Love says: "There is a way. I have traveled it thousands of times."
The intellect saw a market and started to haggle;
Love saw thousands of markets beyond that market.

-Rumi

Alternative Sweetener	Amount of Sugar in Recipe	Amount of Alternative to Use
Agave, Organic Blue**	For 1 cup sugar	Substitute ½ cup to ¾ cup agave and reduce the liquid in recipe by ¼ cup. *Use while transitioning from refined sugars and consider switching to yacon or other alternatives as noted on page 92.*
Amasake*	N/A	Commonly enjoyed as a beverage. Specifics of use are recipe-dependent for vegan and gluten-free baking.

* ** *Please see page 105 for explanatory notes.*

ALTERNATIVE SWEETENER	AMOUNT OF SUGAR IN RECIPE	AMOUNT OF ALTERNATIVE TO USE
BARLEY MALT** *May contain gluten.*	For 1 cup sugar	Substitute 1 to 1½ cups barley malt and reduce liquid in recipe by ¼ cup. Add ¼ tsp baking soda for each cup barley malt used. *Use while transitioning from refined sugars and consider switching to brown rice syrup or yacon syrup or other alternatives as noted on page 92.*
BROWN RICE SYRUP* *If gluten sensitive, look for a gluten-free version, without barley.*	To substitute for liquid sweeteners (e.g. honey, corn syrup, barley malt, agave, or sorghum syrup) For 1 cup sugar	Substitute 1: 1 (e.g. 1 Tbsp of other sweetener for 1 Tbsp brown rice syrup). If using brown rice syrup powder, substitute 1¼ cup for 1 cup of refined sugar and use ¼ cup less of another liquid used in the recipe.
CAROB, OR CAROB SYRUP*	For 1 part cocoa	Substitute 2 ½ parts carob powder (by weight).
CHICOLIN® **	N/A	Is often used combined in small amounts with stevia. Specifics of use are recipe-dependent for vegan and gluten-free baking. *Check with your healthcare practitioner before using this product during your transitional steps.*

* **   *Please see page 105 for explanatory notes.*

ALTERNATIVE SWEETENER	AMOUNT OF SUGAR IN RECIPE	AMOUNT OF ALTERNATIVE TO USE
COCONUT SUGAR*	For 1 cup sugar	Substitute ¾ cup coconut sugar for 1 cup of sugar when using a granular coconut sugar. Can be substituted 1:1 for brown sugar. Substitute coconut sugar (which has a low-glycemic index) for maple sugar crystals in any recipe. *Because coconut sugar is processed by small companies in small batches, flavor may vary from batch to batch. Experimentation with individual results may vary.*
DATE SUGAR*	For 1 cup sugar	Substitute 1:1 if using a granular date sugar. If preparing a date paste from soaked dates, less liquid may be needed. *Individual results may vary.*
DRIED CANE JUICE** *Sometimes called "Dehydrated organic sugar cane juice", "Dried organic cane juice", "Cane juice crystals" or "Evaporated cane juice".*	For 1 cup sugar or brown sugar	Substitute 1 cup Rapadura® or Sucanat®;use a coffee grinder to make a finer crystal. *I recommend Rapadura®. Use while transitioning from refined sugars and consider switching to Rapadura® or other alternatives as noted on page 92.*

* ****** *Please see page 105 for explanatory notes.*

Alternative Sweetener	Amount of Sugar in Recipe	Amount of Alternative to Use
ERYTHRITOL** *May be corn-derived; check with manufacturer.*	For 1 cup sugar	Substitute with 1 cup erythritol or split the recipe between erythritol and maple or coconut sugar crystals.
FLORIDA CRYSTALS®**	For 1 cup sugar	Substitute 1 cup Florida Crystals®
FROZEN FRUIT CONCENTRATE* *If using fruits in recipes, the amount of replacement sweetener will depend on the recipe and the type of fruits used.*	For 1 cup sugar	Substitute with 1 cup frozen fruit concentrate. Recommend blending whole fruit into a paste. *Amount needed will vary, depending upon the recipe. Choosing the whole fruit will provide additional nutrients and fiber not obtained through the concentrate.*
FRUIT, FRESH*	For 1 cup sugar	Individual results may vary based on fruits used and consistency needed.

* ** *Please see page 105 for explanatory notes.*

Alternative Sweetener	Amount of Sugar in Recipe	Amount of Alternative to Use
Fruitsource®*	N/A	Not available for commercial use.
Honey**	For 1 cup sugar	Substitute ½ cup honey and reduce the liquid in recipe by ¼ cup. *Use while transitioning from refined sugars and consider switching to yacon or other alternatives as noted on page 92.*
Jerusalem artichoke syrup*	For 1 cup sugar	For best results, combine this syrup with brown rice syrup or yacon syrup. Substitute ½ cup to ¾ cup combined syrup and reduce the liquid in recipe by ¼ cup. *Some experimentation may be necessary for each recipe.*
Katemfe plant fruit*	N/A	Can be used similar to lo han kuo or stevia in recipes; very little needed (e.g. in quantities of ½ tsp or less).

* ** *Please see page 105 for explanatory notes.*

Alternative Sweetener	Amount of Sugar in Recipe	Amount of Alternative to Use
LAKANTO®**	For 1 cup sugar	Substitute 1 cup Lakanto®
LICORICE ROOT*	N/A	Can be used similar to stevia in recipes; very little needed (e.g. in quantities of ½ tsp or less). *Do not exceed 200 milligrams.*
LO HAN KUO*	N/A	Can be used similar to stevia in recipes; very little needed (e.g. in quantities of ½ tsp or less).
LUCUMA POWDER*	N/A	Though less sweet, can be used similar to stevia in recipes; very little needed (e.g. in quantities of ½ tsp or less).
MAPLE SUGAR CRYSTALS/ PURE MAPLE SYRUP*	For 1 cup sugar	Substitute with 1 cup sugar crystals or syrup. If using liquid syrup, reduce liquid in the recipe by ¼ cup. *Recipe may reach your desired sweetness using less sweetener. If so, adjust the wet and dry ingredients accordingly.*

* **   *Please see page 105 for explanatory notes.*

ALTERNATIVE SWEETENER	AMOUNT OF SUGAR IN RECIPE	AMOUNT OF ALTERNATIVE TO USE
MOLASSES*	For 1 cup sugar	Substitute with 1 cup molasses and reduce liquid in the recipe by ¼ cup. *Recipe may reach your desired sweetness using less molasses. If so, adjust the wet and dry ingredients accordingly.*
RAPADURA®*	For 1 cup sugar	Substitute 1 cup Rapadura®.
SORGHUM SYRUP**	For 1 cup sugar	Substitute with 1 cup sorghum syrup and reduce liquid in the recipe by ¼ cup. *Recipe may reach your desired sweetness using less sorghum. If so, adjust the wet and dry ingredients accordingly. Use while transitioning from refined sugars and consider switching to yacon or other alternatives as noted on page 92.*

* **   *Please see page 105 for explanatory notes.*

Alternative Sweetener	Amount of Sugar in Recipe	Amount of Alternative to Use
STEVIA® * ***	For 1 cup sugar	Powder: ½ - 1 tsp Liquid: 1 tsp
	For 1 Tbsp sugar	Powder: ¼ tsp Liquid: 6-9 drops
	For 1 tsp sugar	Powder: a pinch or 1/16 tsp Liquid: 2-4 drops
		Individual results may vary by recipe.
SUCANAT® **	For 1 cup sugar	Substitute 1 cup Sucanat®.
TAPIOCA SYRUP*	To substitute for liquid sweeteners (e.g. honey, corn syrup, barley malt, agave, or sorghum syrup).	Substitute 1:1 (e.g. 1 Tbsp of other liquid sweetener for 1 Tbsp tapioca syrup).
XYLITOL* *Some varieties may be corn-derived. Only purchase xylitol products with labels noting "made from birch."*	For 1 cup sugar	Substitute with 1 cup xylitol or split the recipe between xylitol and maple or coconut sugar crystals. Xylitol is much sweeter than pure maple syrup. *If using xylitol, I recommend using less than the quantity of pure maple syrup; e.g. less than 1 cup of combined sweeteners.*

* ** ***   *Please see page 105 for explanatory notes.*

ALTERNATIVE SWEETENER	AMOUNT OF SUGAR IN RECIPE	AMOUNT OF ALTERNATIVE TO USE
YACON SYRUP*	For 1 cup sugar	Substitute ½ cup to ¾ cup syrup and reduce the liquid in recipe by ¼ cup. *Some experimentation may be necessary for each recipe.*

* *See page 92 for my recommendations of sweeteners to use with less health risk (as of the printing of this edition). Please see descriptions on pages 74-90 for more details.*

** *Either omit this sweetener or use occasionally in small amounts (one tablespoon or less). Transitional times will vary between individuals. I suggest that people avoid transitional sweeteners altogether (if possible) and experiment with recommended sweeteners instead. Please note that these transitional sweeteners will affect blood sugar in variable amounts. See the descriptions on pages 74-90 for more details.*

*** *Stevia is difficult to use with consistent results in vegan and gluten-free baking. I recommend using it in the recipes where it is noted. Stevia is safe for diabetics and people with candida. Not all brands of stevia are the same. See the Appendix and Resource section on page 296 for quality stevia sources.*

CHAPTER 14

Common

Substitutions for Dairy-, Egg-, Gluten-Free and Vegan Baking

*Everything comes to us that belongs to us,
if we create the capacity to receive it.*

-Tagore

INGREDIENT	DAIRY-, EGG- OR GLUTEN-FREE ALTERNATIVE
Baking mix, traditional (3 cups)	2 cups brown rice flour, ⅔ cup potato starch and ⅓ cup tapioca flour. Yields 3 cups. Store mixture in airtight container. *Potato starch is different from potato flour.* *When using this mix in recipes, you may wish to add baking powder or baking soda (for leavening) to create a delicious final product.* *Please see the Appendix and Resources section on pages 297-298 for suggestions of commercially-prepared gluten-free baking mixes.*

Ingredient	Dairy-, Egg- or Gluten-Free Alternative
Baking powder (1 tsp) *If you prefer to purchase baking powder, but are sensitive to gluten or corn, select a product that is gluten- and corn-free.*	¼ tsp baking soda and ½ tsp cream of tartar, OR 2 parts cream of tartar, 1 part baking soda, 2 parts arrowroot powder
Binding or thickening agent	Xanthan gum (usually corn-derived) ¼ - 1 tsp for cookies (often none is needed) ½ -1 tsp for cakes ¾ tsp for muffins and quick bread 1 - 2 tsp for bread 1 - 2 tsp for pizza crusts Guar gum (corn-free) Chia seeds (used as suggested on page 152) Ground psyllium (can help with thickening or binding in certain recipes) *Measurements vary by recipe and desired final result.*

Ingredient	Dairy-, Egg- or Gluten-Free Alternative
Butter (1 cup)	⅞ cup oil or Organic Earth Balance® (EB). EB has numerous varieties, including soy-free and organic (containing soy). *Both of these varieties are made from corn and contain safflower and canola oils.* OR Virgin coconut oil (amount varies by recipe)
Buttermilk (1 cup)	1 cup dairy-free milk with 1½ Tbsp lemon juice or vinegar
Chocolate, baking (1 square)	3 Tbsp unsweetened, dairy-free cocoa or cacao plus 1 Tbsp Earth Balance®. EB has numerous varieties, including soy-free and organic (containing soy). *Both of these varieties are made from corn and contain safflower and canola oils.*
Egg white (1)	Dissolve 1 Tbsp agar powder in 1 Tbsp filtered water. Whip, then chill in refrigerator and then whip again. *Agar powder is different from agar flakes. For every teaspoon of agar powder, substitute one tablespoon of agar flakes.* OR 1 Tbsp meringue powder plus 2 Tbsp warm filtered water.

Ingredient	Dairy-, Egg- or Gluten-Free Alternative
Egg, whole (1)	1 Tbsp ground flax seed plus ⅛ cup warm filtered water. OR 1 tsp ground chia seeds, ground in coffee grinder with ⅛ cup warm filtered water. Combine these ingredients and allow them to sit for a couple of minutes before adding them to the recipe. OR Commercially-prepared egg replacer. *Follow instructions as noted on product container. I've found that adding egg replacers in my gluten-free recipes, sometimes results in an end product with a more gritty texture.* OR ¼ cup unsweetened applesauce plus ½ tsp aluminum-free baking powder. OR ¼ cup pureéd bananas plus ½ tsp aluminum-free baking powder, OR 1 Tbsp apple cider vinegar
Gelatin	Agar or kudzu/kuzu (*Each recipe is a little different.*)
Shortening or Crisco® (1 cup)	⅔ cup oil, OR 1 cup Earth Balance® shortening

Ingredient	Dairy-, Egg- or Gluten-Free Alternative
Wheat flour (1 cup)	Wheat-free alternatives: 1 ¼ cups barley flour 1 cup kamut flour 1 ¼ cups rye flour 1 cup spelt flour Gluten-free alternatives: 1¼ cups oat flour (*see* Appendix and Resources *section on page 298 for gluten-free brands*) 1¼ cups rice flour 1 cup teff flour ¾ cup quinoa flour plus ¼ cup arrowroot or tapioca starch ¾ cup amaranth flour plus ¼ cup arrowroot or tapioca starch ¾ cup buckwheat flour plus ¼ cup arrowroot or tapioca starch ¾ cup chickpea (garbanzo) flour plus ¼ cup arrowroot or tapioca starch 1 cup rice flour plus ¼ cup tapioca flour plus ¼ cup nut flour 2 cups brown rice flour, ⅔ cup potato starch and ⅓ cup tapioca flour. Yields 3 cups. Store mixture in airtight container. *Potato starch is different from potato flour.* continued

Ingredient	Dairy-, Egg- or Gluten-Free Alternative
Wheat flour (1 cup) (continued)	*Though a variety of other gluten-free and wheat-free flour substitutes are available (i.e. soy flour, bean flours, corn flour, etc.), they are not listed here because they may cause discomfort for people with food allergies.*

Beverages

Bon Bons

Cakes

Cookies

PART 2

The Recipes

Frozen

I am very excited to share these recipes with you. Our family had a wonderful time making these goodies. I hope that you enjoy making them, eating them, and sharing them, and that you will love them as much as we have.

Muffins

I look forward to hearing your stories and thoughts.

Smoothies

Many of these recipes are pictured on my website: *www.SweetnessWithoutSugar.com*

Raw

Author's Notes, Suggestions and Tips

Complete health and awakening are really the same.

-Tarthang Tulku

These recipes were written with the idea that many who are trying them will be "coming off of sugar" and are used to a very sweet taste. If you are transitioning from sugar to alternative sweeteners, and/or have already omitted artificial sweeteners and sugar from your diet, you may enjoy these recipes with even less sweetener than noted in the recipes.

Choosing a sweetener depends on personal taste, health challenges, your desire for whole food and your possible need for low-glycemic foods. Although these recipes have some variations noted, they have been tested to taste good as written and analyzed. In most cases, I chose to offer nutritional analyses for the recipes with the highest levels of sweetness. This way you can make conscious choices and alter the recipes to your current eating habits. Remember that recipes with higher amounts of sweetener also contain healthy proteins, fats and other nutrients. This way, you may choose to have a smaller serving size than what is noted, or make changes according to your personal preferences.

Although using alternative sweeteners is a step above sugar and artificial sweeteners, it is not a prescription to eat as much as you may like. Low glycemic alternatives such as stevia, yacon syrup, xylitol and maple sugar crystals (in small amounts) often make the best choices.

Perhaps you want to consume only natural, unprocessed and wholesome sweeteners. Some examples to try include stevia, date paste, raw honey, or puréed fruits. People can still have food sensitivities and blood sugar reactions to alternative sweeteners. I invite you to trust your body and be aware of any symptoms you experience after trying different sweeteners.

Just because an item is found in a health food store or in a "healthy sweetener" aisle does not mean it is the choice that is best for you. My goal is to provide you with enough information to make educated choices. Sometimes a nutritional consultation can help navigate your personal needs. Please contact me for further recommendations.

Although I acknowledge a rise in nut sensitivities and include information about this in this book, there are also recipes included here that contain nuts.

These "nut recipes" also work well with seed butters (e.g. sunflower seed, pumpkin seed, hempseed) and other nut butters except for those made from peanuts or tree nuts. Even if you or your family can tolerate nuts, if you choose to make these recipes for a party or a school event, you can substitute with a seed butter if desired.

I use almonds and/or almond meal/flour in a number of recipes too. Almonds are slightly sweet, alkalizing nuts (especially when soaked) that can add satiety, healthy fat (when consumed in moderation), magnesium, minerals and a little bit of protein. Due to the natural toxin found in peanuts (e.g. aflatoxin), I recommend choosing from the wide array of other nut butters available on the market today. Nutritional analyses for recipes containing nuts, seeds, and oils may indicate higher amounts of fat than other recipes. As mentioned in Chapter 7 on *Essential Fatty Acids* on pages 35-40, not all fat is created equal.

For your convenience, I have included an allergen-free guide after the directions for each recipe. Because the whole book is dairy-, egg-, gluten- and wheat-free, I've highlighted other common allergens including nuts, seeds, corn and/or soy. If nut- or seed-free is indicated on a recipe, the recipe can be made *either* nut- or seed-free, but not both. This "at-a-glance" guide can be handy when preparing recipes for people with different food sensitivities or allergies.

Sea salt contains minerals which are usually stripped from Kosher and table salts. I recommend using Celtic sea salt, and/or Himalayan crystal salt, though more expensive, because they contain the most minerals and trace elements. Other commercially-prepared sea salts may lack vital minerals. In general, one can use a smaller quantity of sea salt than traditional table salt to achieve the same effect.

Aluminum-free baking powder is recommended because aluminum has been linked in research to a higher incidence of Alzheimer's Disease. If your baking powder is not labeled as aluminum-free, it likely contains aluminum. *Most commercial baking powders (even aluminum-free brands) contain cornstarch. If you are sensitive to corn, consider making your own baking powder. For baking powder substitutions, see page 108.*

In baked or raw recipes, I replaced eggs and dairy with vegan protein sources because both eggs and dairy foods are common food allergens for many people. Dairy foods also generally contain higher amounts of sugar. Consequently, the recipes here include protein sources like brown rice, hemp and raw protein powders.

If you have trouble locating ingredients, many can be found at (or special ordered from) your local health food stores, through websites and sources noted in the *Appendix and Resources* section on pages 293-317, through my website, or by contacting me. Many standard grocery stores now have "health food sections" where some of these items are available packaged and/or in the bulk bin food section.

Another point of interest related to these products is their cost. Gluten-free flours and superfood products are more expensive. If you are living on a budget, cost is a factor to consider. When I work with people, I advise they buy small quantities of items (e.g. from the bulk food section of a grocery store) to test their tolerance to these foods. Superfoods are often sold in different sizes, so beginning with a trial size is a great way for you and your loved ones to test the product.

The ingredients used in this section provide nutrients our bodies need. When replacing nutrient-deficient ingredients with these healthful ingredients, our bodies change and feel satiated with smaller quantities, resulting in better health. I believe that if people miss less work, have more energy, feel better, and visit the doctor less, then the money spent on these ingredients is worthwhile.

Unfortunately, our culture makes it affordable to buy foods containing additives, excitotoxins, processed ingredients, corn syrup and other manufactured ingredients. This occurs because those foods are produced using inexpensive, surplus ingredients, not because the ingredients are healthier for us to consume.

Though I do not explicitly specify using organic fruits and vegetables, I recommend using produce free of harmful pesticides, herbicides and fungicides whenever possible. For your convenience, I've included a list (on page 120) highlighting the most commonly sprayed produce (highest in pesticides). When your budget allows, at least choose organic versions of these fruits and vegetables. Certified organic foods are grown without genetically-modified ingredients and will optimize your health.

As consumers begin to seek healthier, organic foods, many large manufacturers have begun to produce healthy product lines. This practice has led large companies to purchase smaller companies, resulting in a wide array of products. The J.M. Smucker Company® owns R.W. Knudsen Family®, which sells juice drinks and fruit-sweetened spreads. The Hershey Company® owns Dagoba® Organic Chocolate, a product that contains a high cacao content and is mostly found in health food stores.

I advocate choosing products that nourish
both our bodies and our planet.

When we purchase Dagoba® chocolate, we support the larger company that produces foods containing high fructose corn syrup, and in turn, our dollars may contribute to the bigger issue of sugar addiction. On the contrary, if we are selective about the sweeteners we consume and the companies we support, our consumer demand can truly change the structure of our food supply. In most cases, I have suggested products that remain independent. For more information on this subject and to learn which companies remain independent, please contact me.

These recipes were analyzed using Food Processor Nutrition & Fitness Software from ESHA Research (version 10.2.3), 2008. If the daily value percentages of vitamin A, C, calcium, or iron did not apply, they were not listed. Though the recipes in this book are all cholesterol and trans-fat free, cholesterol and trans-fat are noted in the analyses because many people are interested in that information for health reasons. Other nutrients with a zero value were not listed in the analyses.

In most cases, the recipes were analyzed using quantities with the highest amount of sweetener most likely available in stores. For instance, many recipes were analyzed using pure maple syrup or brown rice syrup rather than yacon syrup. If the recipe suggests adding "½ cup to 1 cup of sweetener", the recipe was analyzed at the 1 cup value.

This allows you the option to eat the whole portion as listed, to eat a smaller portion and/or to create the recipe with an alternative sweetener that is not as sweet. Having a range is part of the sweetness journey.

The sweet snacks and desserts noted in this book are not only delicious, but they contain protein, calcium and essential fatty acids. I hope that you notice a difference in the way you feel when eating these treats. As mentioned previously, indulging our sweet tooth with healthy treats is a way to nourish ourselves and our cells. The spectrum of healthy is an individual journey. Trust where you are now and use your intuition to help guide you. Even if you overindulge, ridding your body of artificial sweeteners and refined sugar will greatly enhance your life.

I strongly suggest that we value our health and well-being now more than ever. We can show our enthusiasm by supporting our local growers, reducing our use of fossil fuels and purchasing products made from wholesome ingredients produced closest to where we live. If we want change, we have a choice to make changes for ourselves. As the infamous Nelson Mandela has said: *"Be the change you wish to see in the world."* Each step counts and makes a difference.

All of these recipes have been both kid- and adult-approved. I hope that you enjoy them!

> *It is never too late to be what you might have been.*
> — George Elliot

Pesticides and Conventional Produce: Making Wise Choices*

High Pesticide Foods

Apples
Apricots
Bell peppers
Blackberries
Blueberries
Cantaloupes (Mexican higher than US)
Carrots
Celery

Cherries (US higher than imported cherries)
Cotton
Grapes
Green beans
Kale
Lettuce
Nectarines

Peaches
Pears
Potatoes
Red raspberries
Spinach
Strawberries
Watermelon
Winter squash

Low Pesticide Foods

Asparagus
Avocado
Bananas
Blackberries
Broccoli
Brussels sprouts
Cabbage
Cauliflower
Citrus fruits
Corn (frozen too)

Cucumbers
Eggplant
Grapefruit
Hemp
Honeydew
Kiwi fruit
Mangos
Onions
Papayas

Peas (green, sweet) (frozen too)
Pineapples
Plums
Scallions (green onions)
Sweet potatoes
Radishes
Romaine lettuce
Tomatoes
Watermelon

Sources:

www.assatashakur.org/forum/showthread.php?t=2657

Environmental Working Group's Food News (www.foodnews.org)*

---

* *Visit www.foodnews.org for a "Shopper's Guide to Pesticides" magnet or convenient wallet guide.*

Beverages

When preparing these beverages or filling your daily water bottles or glasses, consider adding a personalized sentence, word, or message such as "Love", "Health", "Compassion", "I am healthy and vibrant" or whatever you choose. Tape messages so they face inward, toward the contents of the bottle (as if the liquid inside can read the message). If you wish, tape the same message outward, so you can read it too! This simple action has been shown to benefit our health in amazing ways. To read more on this stunning research, you may wish to read The Hidden Messages in Water or The True Power of Water by Masaru Emoto.

Many of these recipes are pictured on my website: *www.SweetnessWithoutSugar.com*

LAVENDER CHAMOMILE WATER

A nice refreshing and relaxing beverage. Sometimes our sugar cravings indicate a need to slow down and get away from the "to do lists." This is a nice beverage that will help you "take a breather." It can serve as a mini meditation time or break to share alone or with your children. This drink can be steeped for as long as you like, to suit your taste and temperature preferences.

4 Tbsp organic and/or biodynamically grown lavender

4 cups filtered water

1. Combine lavender and water in a bell jar or glass container. Cover and set in the sun or, during the winter months, in a warm room. *As an alternative, and to save time, try using a French press.*

2. Let this combination sit overnight or up to 24 hours (*less if you prefer a lighter taste*).

3. Pour the lavender water through a tea strainer or colander. Capture the liquid in a pitcher or glass container. Discard the lavender. *If using a French press, push the plunger down, drink the liquid while discarding the lavender.*

4. Drink within 3-4 days. Adjust the amount of lavender to suit your preference.

Makes: 4 cups
Preparation time: 5 minutes
Steeping time: 8 to 24 hours
Serving size: 1 cup

Corn-Free | Nut and Seed-Free | Nut or Seed-Free | Soy-Free

HINTS, TIPS AND SUBSTITUTIONS

You may want to substitute chamomile for lavender. Or, for a nice, calming blend that is great warmed for kids, combine 2 tablespoons lavender with 2 tablespoons chamomile. To make the flavor more subtle, add a little water or sparkling mineral water. If desired, add stevia to taste.

This recipe can be enjoyed if you are following a raw diet. For more raw recipes, please see pages 247-291.

AMOUNT PER 1 CUP SERVING: Calories 5; Calories from Fat 0; Total Fat 0g; Saturated Fat 0g; Trans Fat 0g; Cholesterol 0mg; Sodium 10mg; Total Carbohydrate 1g; Dietary Fiber 0g; Sugars 0g; Protein 0g. *Recipe analyzed with chamomile and filtered spring water.*

SPICED "MILK"

Refreshing yet with warming spices, this nice, blended treat provides protein and healthy fat. It's also a soothing, warmed drink before bedtime, on a cold morning or during a cold wintry day.

2 cups unsweetened, dairy-free milk (e.g. almond, brown rice or hemp milk)

¼ tsp cinnamon

¼ tsp cardamom

1-2 Tbsp coconut *cream* (not oil, optional)

12 or less drops of liquid stevia to taste

1. Combine all ingredients and warm over medium-low heat for 5-7 minutes.

2. Pour into a mug and enjoy.

Makes: 2 cups
Preparation time: 5 - 10 minutes
Serving size: 1 cup

Corn-Free | *Nut and Seed-Free* | *Nut or Seed-Free* | *Soy-Free*

HINTS, TIPS AND SUBSTITUTIONS

For a raw version of this recipe, please see page 250.

AMOUNT PER 1 CUP SERVING: Calories 160; Calories from Fat 110; Total Fat 12g; Saturated Fat 5g; Trans Fat 0g; Cholesterol 0mg; Sodium 25mg; Total Carbohydrate 2g; Dietary Fiber 2g; Sugars 0g; Protein 6g; Iron 20% DV; Calcium 2% DV. *Recipe analyzed with unsweetened Hemp Bliss Original® hemp milk and 2 Tbsp coconut cream.*

HOT CHOCOLATE

Having met many people with fond memories of drinking hot chocolate during the winter, I've provided this tasty, healthy version for those stormy days when you want to sip it by the fireplace.

1 cup unsweetened, dairy-free milk (e.g. almond, brown rice or hemp milk)

1 Tbsp, slightly heaping, unsweetened, dairy-free cocoa powder

¼ tsp ground cinnamon

1 small vanilla bean (ground in coffee grinder) or split in half (or ½ tsp alcohol-free vanilla flavoring)

Pinch of nutmg and/or cloves or cardamom

4-6 drops liquid stevia (to your taste; use a flavored stevia if preferred)

1. Combine all ingredients into a saucepan and bring the contents to a slight boil.

2. Stir the ingredients continuously for 5-7 minutes, until hot. Serve and enjoy!

Makes: 1 cup
Preparation time: 10 minutes
Serving size: 1 cup

Corn-Free* | *Nut and Seed-Free* | *Nut or Seed-Free* | *Soy-Free*

* Check labels

HINTS, TIPS AND SUBSTITUTIONS

See the Appendix and Resources *section on page 306 for dairy-free cocoa suggestions.*

Use So Delicous® Coconut Creamer for added creaminess, flavor and richness.

If you are following a raw diet, you may enjoy this recipe warm (see page 251). For more raw recipes, please see pages 247-291.

AMOUNT PER 1 CUP SERVING: Calories 140; Calories from Fat 70; Total Fat 8g; Saturated Fat 1g; Trans Fat 0g; Cholesterol 0mg; Sodium 25mg; Total Carbohydrate 5g; Dietary Fiber 3g; Sugars 0g; Protein 6g; Calcium 2%DV; Iron 25%DV. *Recipe analyzed with* Hemp Bliss Unsweetened® *Original hemp milk and without coconut creamer.*

HOMEMADE YOGI TEA

Although this is not an original recipe, it is one we often have in our home that appeals to many tastes. I have taken out the actual "tea" (usually a black tea is added at the end) and have enjoyed a "tea" of herbs. Handling the beautiful herbs with our children is a fun and easy activity we share. They also like to drink this tea with our family.

3 quarts filtered water

24 whole black peppercorns (about ½ tsp)

24 whole green cardamom pods (about ¾ Tbsp)

18 whole cloves (about 1 tsp)

5 cinnamon sticks

2½ inches of peeled and sliced ginger root (about 1½ Tbsp)

6 whole stars of star anise (can also use 1 level Tbsp fenugreek seeds)

1½ tsp black tea (can use decaf; or omit) (1 tea bag)

1 quart (if desired) unsweetened, dairy-free milk (e.g. almond, brown rice or hemp milk)

Liquid stevia to taste

1. Bring the water to a boil and add all of the above ingredients except for the tea, milk and stevia.

2. Allow the mixture to simmer for 30 minutes. Then turn off heat, add the tea, cover the saucepan, and let it steep for 10 minutes. Steeping for longer than 30 minutes may create a bitter flavor. If you prefer to reheat this tea, omit the black tea. This version is flavorful and yummy. While it simmers, this tea makes the house smell nice.

3. Ladle cupfuls out of the pot or strain the mixture. Add the rice or hemp milk and stevia as desired. Traditionally, the "milk" is added once the tea has brewed. Serve this warm or cold (in summer).

Makes: 3 quarts (12 cups)
Preparation time: 10 minutes
Steeping/boiling time: 30 minutes
Serving size: 1 cup

Corn-Free* | *Nut and Seed-Free* | *Nut or Seed-Free* | *Soy-Free*

* Check labels

AMOUNT PER 1 CUP SERVING: Calories 40; Calories from Fat 20; Total Fat 2.5g; Saturated Fat 0g; Trans Fat 0g; Cholesterol 0mg; Sodium 20mg; Total Carbohydrate 2g; Dietary Fiber 1g; Sugars 0g; Protein 2g; Calcium 2% DV; Iron 8% DV. *Recipe analyzed with Hemp Bliss® unsweetened hemp milk and black tea. Our family normally omits the black tea.*

Adding a little fresh orange peel makes
it smell and taste wonderful.

SPARKLING WATER WITH STEVIA FLAVORS

Since 1978, consumption of soft drinks has more than tripled for boys and doubled for girls. My sparkling drink is a great alternative to soda! With this recipe, you can still enjoy the "bubbles" and sweet flavors reminiscent of soda. There are so many stevia flavors to choose from such as root beer, grape, orange and more. Adding apple juice to sparkling water brings back memories of a trip to England where "appletizers" (a very sweet, carbonated apple drink), were offered in most restaurants.

8 oz. Gerolsteiner® or other sparkling water

Add one of the following:

4 or more drops of flavored stevia

1-2 tsp (2 oz) bottled juice concentrate before reconstituting

(e.g. Woodstock Farms® Pomegranate Juice)

1 orange, 1 apple, or ½ grapefruit (fresh-squeezed)

1. Combine Gerlosteiner® or mineral water with one of the flavorings listed above.

2. Mix well and enjoy. *For extra fun, drink with a straw.*

Makes: 1 cup
Preparation time: 5 minutes
Serving size: 1 cup

Corn-Free | *Nut and Seed-Free* | *Nut or Seed-Free* | *Soy-Free*

HINTS, TIPS AND SUBSTITUTIONS

If you are corn-sensitive and plan to use bottled juice in this recipe, purchase a juice brand that does not contain ascorbic acid.

This recipe can be enjoyed if you are following a raw diet. For more raw recipes, please see pages 247-291.

SPARKLING WATER WITH STEVIA FLAVORS:

AMOUNT PER 1 CUP SERVING: Calories 0; Calories from Fat 0; Total Fat 0g; Saturated Fat 0g; Trans Fat 0g; Cholesterol 0mg; Sodium 30mg; Total Carbohydrate 0g; Dietary Fiber 0g; Sugars 0g; Protein 0g; Calcium 8% DV. *Recipe analyzed with stevia and Gerlosteiner® water.*

SPARKLING WATER WITH POMEGRANATE CONCENTRATE:

AMOUNT PER 1 CUP SERVING: Calories 25; Calories from Fat 0; Total Fat 0g; Saturated Fat 0g; Trans Fat 0g; Cholesterol 0mg; Sodium 30mg; Total Carbohydrate 6g; Dietary Fiber 0g; Sugars 5g; Protein 0g; Calcium 10% DV Iron 2% DV. *Recipe analyzed with Gerlosteiner® and 2 tsp pomegranate concentrate.*

SPARKLING WATER WITH 2 OZ. APPLE JUICE:

AMOUNT PER 1 CUP SERVING: Calories 25; Calories from Fat 0; Total Fat 0g; Saturated Fat 0g; Trans Fat 0g; Cholesterol 0mg; Sodium 30mg; Total Carbohydrate 7g; Dietary Fiber 0g; Sugars 6g; Protein 0g; Calcium 8% DV. *Recipe analyzed with ¼ cup store-bought Lakewood® Apple Juice and Gerlosteiner® water.*

COCONUT KEFIR

Making this drink is worth the effort. Once the coconuts are opened, the rest is easy. Kefir is wonderful for helping to restore gut health and for minimizing sugar and sweet cravings. It will also offer a healthy bacteria perk when you're travelling or in the midst of cold and flu season.

3-4 Thai young coconuts (the white cone-shaped coconuts)

1 packet kefir culture (the Body Ecology® brand works very well)

1. Using a sharp knife, cut slices from the bottom of the coconuts (the flat side) until you see the brown or white ring/soft spot.

2. Using an apple corer, vegetable peeler or small paring knife, poke a hole in the soft spot (the round ring) near or at the location of the brown or white spot. Use a peeler to dig the hole out.

3. Prepare to overturn the coconut and capture the liquid in a measuring cup or glass bell jar. Drain. Set the coconut water aside after making sure it is a light tan/yellow color. Coconut water that is pink in color should be discarded. Repeat these steps with each coconut until you collect one quart of liquid.

4. Add kefir starter culture (purchased from a health food store or online via the link noted under "Hints" on the next page).

5. Cover the quart of liquid and shake it well. For best results, place in a warm room for 2-3 days. Kefir will be ready when small bubbles appear after the container is moved slightly.

6. Enjoy this bubbly, refreshing and healthy drink. If giving kefir to children, start with 1-2 ounces at a time and work up from there to ½ cup.

Makes: 1 quart (4 cups)
Preparation time: 30 minutes or more
Waiting time: 3 days
Serving size: 1 oz. for babies/ ½ cup or more for toddlers/
1 cup for adults

Corn-Free | *Nut and Seed-Free* | *Nut or Seed-Free* | *Soy-Free*

HINTS, TIPS AND SUBSTITUTIONS

To view a description and demonstration of how to make this delicious and healthy drink, visit

www.bodyecology.com/mcoconutkefir.php.

I recommend reviewing this site for details on how to prepare the liquid and scoop out the fresh coconut! Yum! We have had positive results using one packet of kefir culture for two Thai coconuts (without straining or heating beforehand) though the quantity of liquid is less than a full quart.

If you have a strong sensitivity to sugar (e.g. candida, sugar addictions, etc.), you may wish to increase your serving size initially (on an individual basis) or contact me for a consultation.

This recipe can be enjoyed if you are following a raw diet. For more raw recipes, please see pages 247-291.

AMOUNT PER 1 CUP SERVING: Calories 40; Calories from Fat 5;
Total Fat .5g; Saturated Fat 0g; Trans Fat 0g; Cholesterol 0mg;
Sodium 220mg; Total Carbohydrate 8g; Dietary Fiber 2g; Sugars 6g;
Protein 2g; Vitamin C 8% DV; Calcium 4% DV; Iron 4% DV.

When our children were seven months old, we gave them one ounce of kefir per day (as a test, for 3-4 days). Their bodies handled it well and they seemed to love the drink! Our son, Solomon enjoys a 4-6 ounce serving of kefir whenever his immune system needs a little boost.

HOMEMADE NUT OR SEED "MILK"

This easy "milk" recipe was inspired by drinks featured in Laura Bruno's <u>The Lazy Raw Foodist's Guide</u>. Laura's wonderful resource guide (which is for everyone, even non-raw foodists) includes tips and recipe variations. When using the Jack LaLanne Power Elite Juicer®, this "milk" is simple to make!

1-2 cups soaked nuts or seeds

3-6 cups filtered water

2 pitted dates (optional)

Liquid stevia to taste

1. Soak the nuts or seeds in filtered water. (See the chart on page 134 for more information on soaking and sprouting times for nuts and seeds.) Drain.

2. Blend soaked nuts or seeds with new filtered water. Use enough water to create your desired thickness. *Combining three or four parts water to one part nuts will create "milk" most people enjoy. For example, use 1 cup nuts to 3-4 cups of filtered water.*

3. If desired, drink the milk plain. You can also sweeten the milk with enough drops of stevia to suit your taste, or add pitted dates and re-blend.

4. Set aside a big bowl and a sprout bag or cheesecloth. *(Cheesecloth is messier to use.)* Pour the liquid into a sprout bag and drain into bowl. Squeeze the contents to get more liquid out of the "pulp." For a pictorial demonstration of raw nut or milk preparation, visit this link: *www.rawglow.com/almond milkhowto.htm.*

Makes: 3 to 6 cups "milk"
Soaking time: varies 2-12 hours
Blend and strain time: 20 minutes
Serving size: ½ cup toddler, 1 cup adult

Corn-Free | ~~*Nut and Seed-Free*~~ | **Nut or Seed-Free** | *Soy-Free*

HINTS, TIPS AND SUBSTITUTIONS

Use the chart on page 134 to determine soaking time. If soaking time is between 8-12 hours, soaking the nuts/seeds overnight is easiest.

For a raw version of this recipe, please see page 256.

AMOUNT PER 1 CUP SERVING: Calories 300; Calories from Fat 210; Total Fat 24g; Saturated Fat 2g; Trans Fat 0g; Cholesterol 0mg; Sodium 5mg; Total Carbohydrate 16g; Dietary Fiber 6g; Sugars 7g; Protein 10g; Calcium 15% DV; Iron 10% DV. *Recipe analyzed with 2 cups raw, unsalted almonds, 2 dates and 6 cups water.*

A Soaking and Sprouting Chart
for Nuts and Seeds

Item	Dry Measure	Soaking Water Temperature	Soaking Time	Sprouting Time
NUTS				
Almonds	1 cup	Cool-Warm	12 hours	3 days
Brazil nuts			Do not soak	N/A
Cashews			Do not soak	N/A
Macadamia			Do not soak	N/A
Pecans	1 cup	Cool-Warm	2-4 hours	N/A
Pine Nuts			Do not soak	N/A
Pistachio, in shell			Do not soak	N/A
Walnuts	1 cup	Warm	2-4 hours	N/A
SEEDS				
Chia seeds	1 cup	Cool	2-4 hours	2-4 hours up to 3 days
Flax seeds			Do not soak	N/A
Hempseeds			Do not soak	N/A
Pumpkin seeds	1 cup	Cool	4-8 hours	24 hours up to 3 days
Sesame seeds, Black	1 cup	Cool	4 hours	N/A
Sesame seeds, White Hulled	1 cup	Cool	4 hours	N/A
Sunflower seeds, hulled	1 cup	Cool	4-8 hours	24 hours

References:

❋ *Conscious Eating* by Gabriel Cousens, MD.
❋ *Rainbow Green Live-Food Cuisine* by Gabriel Cousens, MD.
❋ *Nourishing Traditions* by Sally Fallon.
❋ *Healing with Whole Foods* by Paul Pitchford.

Bon Bons
and Truffles

 Many of these recipes are pictured on my
website: *www.SweetnessWithoutSugar.com*

NUT BALLS

This recipe, inspired by Dr. Joseph Mercola, was once referred to as halvah. But when a dear friend repeatedly asked me to bring "those nut balls" to our get-togethers, the "nut ball" name stuck. Since then, many new versions of nut balls have emerged. All freeze well and can stay in the refrigerator for up to two weeks in an airtight container (if they aren't gobbled up before then!)

½ cup ground walnuts, almonds, cashews or pecans, (ground in coffee grinder or blender with a dry blade attachment) or use store-bought flours (e.g. almond meal or hazelnut flour)

½ cup unsweetened, unsulphured, shredded organic coconut

¼ plus ⅛ cup Nutribiotic® Rice Protein or hemp protein, or ¾ cup (1½ scoops) Sun Warrior Protein®

½ cup unsalted and unsweetened almond, cashew or sesame butter (e.g. almond butter or tahini)

¼ cup unsweetened organic canned coconut milk (use more or less to suit your taste and consistency preferences) or fresh coconut cream.

½ cup dried blueberries (unsweetened, corn syrup- and sugar-free)

6-10 Tbsp brown rice syrup or yacon or 5 drops liquid stevia (or to taste)

1. Combine all ingredients in a bowl. Can use a coffee grinder or a dry blade to grind nuts into a fine powder.

2. Use a spoon to mix until the combination stays together. (*Add more coconut milk to suit your taste and texture preferences.*)

3. Scoop into balls using a heaping teaspoon.

4. These can be served immediately or stored in the refrigerator (if they aren't eaten before they get to the refrigerator). If desired, sprinkle with coconut shreds or raw cacao. These also store well in the freezer.

Makes: 32 balls
Preparation time: 15 minutes
Serving size: 2 balls

Corn-Free | ~~*Nut and Seed-Free*~~ | **Nut or Seed-Free** | *Soy-Free*

HINTS, TIPS AND SUBSTITUTIONS

If you are sensitive to nuts, try sunflower or pumpkin seeds.

For those needing a little extra sweetness, consider adding a drop of stevia to the outside of the ball before eating. Coat it with your fingers to evenly distribute the sweet flavor.

Consider doubling this recipe. They'll go fast!

For a raw version of this recipe, please see page 258.

AMOUNT PER 2 BALL SERVING: Calories 170; Calories from Fat 90; Total Fat 10g; Saturated Fat 3g; Trans Fat 0g; Cholesterol 0mg; Sodium 25mg; Total Carbohydrate 15g; Dietary Fiber 2g; Sugars 8g; Protein 7g; Calcium 2% DV; Iron 6% DV; Calcium 2% DV. *Recipe analyzed using pecans, tahini, Nutribiotic® brown rice protein and 8 Tbsp brown rice syrup.*

These healthy treats contain omega fats, protein
and other nutrients, and always provide sweet
smiles. One serving is quite satisfying.

TAHINI ORANGE TURKISH TAFFY

Here is a way to have taffy without it sticking to your teeth. The delicious flavor continues to unfold in your mouth. It is also packed with protein and fiber.

½ cup unsalted and unsweetened tahini

¾ cup packed chopped soaked dates (when chopped and pressed down,
   they measure ¾c)

½ cup water from soaked dates

2 tsp minced ginger

2 tsp orange peel (zest)

1 tsp alcohol-free orange flavoring

½ cup (2 scoops) Sun Warrior Natural Protein®

5-9 tsp psyllium husk powder

Liquid stevia to taste

1. Blend tahini, soaked dates and water, ginger, orange peel, orange flavor and protein powder in a Cuisinart® or blender.

2. Gradually add up to five teaspoons of psyllium (one teaspoon at a time) and blend after each addition, until mixture is smooth, but firm enough to form into balls.

3. Let the mixture sit for up to 15 minutes. If necessary, add more psyllium. Psyllium takes a little time to fully absorb.

4. Use a teaspoon to form into balls. Chill taffy balls in the refrigerator or freezer.

Makes: Approx. 20 pieces
Preparation time: 20 minutes
Serving size: 2 pieces

Corn-Free | ~~Nut and Seed-Free~~ | **Nut or Seed-Free** | **Soy-Free**

HINTS, TIPS AND SUBSTITUTIONS

You can also use Nutribiotic® Vanilla Rice Protein, and add more stevia to the finished taffy for extra flavor.

For a raw version of this recipe, please see page 260.

AMOUNT PER 2 PIECE SERVING: Calories 130; Calories from Fat 70; Total Fat 8g; Saturated Fat 1g; Trans Fat 0g; Cholesterol 0mg; Sodium 15mg; Total Carbohydrate 13g; Dietary Fiber 2g; Sugars 9g; Protein 7g; Vitamin A 2% DV; Vitamin C 2% DV; Calcium 4% DV; Iron 10% DV. *Recipe analyzed with non-raw sesame butter and nine teaspoons psyllium husk powder.*

GOJI GO BON BONS

These provide high-quality protein, absorbable greens, fiber and antioxidants. They are easy to take with you for travel, lunches, snacks and picnics. Even those who aren't fans of the goji taste will enjoy the subtle flavors of this healthy bon bon.

1 cup unsalted and unsweetened almond or hempseed butter

⅛ cup (½ scoop) Sun Warrior Protein®, any flavor

⅛ cup or 2 Tbsp hemp protein powder

¼ cup ground goji berries (ground in coffee grinder)

½ tsp spirulina powder

1 tsp acai powder

¼ cup ground flax seed (ground in coffee grinder)

¼ cup brown rice syrup or yacon syrup or liquid stevia to taste

For rolling or outer coating:

Ground goji berries

Hempseeds

Unsweetened, unsulphured, shredded organic coconut

Cacao nibs (whole or ground in coffee grinder - to your preference)

1. Combine all ingredients in a medium-sized bowl.

2. Use your hands to shape the mixture into teaspoon-sized balls.

3. Roll balls to coat them in any of the above options or eat as is.

4. Store in an airtight container in the refrigerator until ready to eat.

Makes: 30 bon bons
Preparation time: 20 minutes
Serving size: 2 bon bons

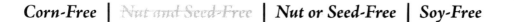

Corn-Free | ~~Nut and Seed-Free~~ | *Nut or Seed-Free* | *Soy-Free*

HINTS, TIPS AND SUBSTITUTIONS

For a raw version of this recipe, please see page 262.

AMOUNT PER 2 BON BON SERVING WITHOUT OUTER COATING: Calories 150; Calories from Fat 100; Total Fat 11g; Saturated Fat 1g; Trans Fat 0g; Cholesterol 0mg; Sodium 95mg; Total Carbohydrate 11g; Dietary Fiber 2g; Sugars 5g; Protein 4g; Calcium 6% DV; Iron 6% DV. *Recipe analyzed with unsalted smooth almond butter and brown rice syrup.*

BROWNIE BON BONS

These tasty bites of chocolate, similar to super soft brownies, get their protein from tofu and "milk". They are quite fun to eat. Good for a special treat in a lunch box.

¼ cup firm organic tofu (boxed or refrigerated)

¼ cup unsweetened, dairy-free milk (e.g. almond, brown rice or hemp milk)

2 Tbsp unsweetened fruit spread of choice

1 Tbsp organic unrefined walnut or sunflower oil

1 tsp alcohol-free vanilla flavoring

¼ cup plus ⅛ cup maple or coconut sugar crystals (ground in coffee grinder)

¼ cup plus ⅛ cup xylitol sweetener (ground in coffee grinder)

⅓ cup unsweetened, dairy-free cocoa powder or carob

½ cup gluten-free flour (e.g. brown rice or millet flour or an all-purpose
      gluten-free mix)

½ tsp aluminum-free baking powder

¼ tsp sea or Himalayan salt

Add nuts and/or fruit-sweetened, allergen- and dairy-free chocolate chips
      or vegan carob chips, if desired. (*These chips may contain cane sugar.*)

1. Preheat oven to 350°F. Lightly grease an 8 x 8 pan with unrefined oil and set aside. Pureé the tofu and dairy-free milk until smooth. Pour this mixture into a bowl.

2. Add the fruit spread, oil, and vanilla to the bowl. Mix, then add in the ground maple sugar crystals, ground xylitol, cocoa powder, flour, baking powder and salt. Mix again.

3. If desired, add nuts or chocolate chips and pour batter into an oiled pan. Smooth the batter to make it even (batter may be thick).

4. Bake at 350°F for 20-25 minutes. *The batter may not rise very much and will remain gooey.*

5. Let the brownies cool. Then spoon into tablespoon-sized balls and roll into bon bons. Can be served with *Cherry Berry Sauce* on page 162.

Makes: 16 bon bons
Preparation time: 30 minutes
Baking time: 20-25 minutes
Serving size: 2 bon bons

Corn-Free* | *Nut and Seed-Free* | *Nut or Seed-Free* | *Soy-Free*

* Check labels

HINTS, TIPS AND SUBSTITUTIONS

If you prefer to use only maple sugar crystals, use ¾ cup or less for the entire recipe.

See the Appendix and Resources section on pages 300-306 for dairy-free cocoa and milk suggestions.

Packaged carob may contain gluten and corn. To make your own carob chips, see page 184 for a stevia-sweetened option.

AMOUNT PER 2 BON BON SERVING: Calories 130; Calories from Fat 25; Total Fat 3g; Saturated Fat 0g; Trans Fat 0g; Cholesterol 0mg; Sodium 170mg; Total Carbohydrate 29g; Dietary Fiber 2g; Sugars 8g; Protein 2g; Calcium 2% DV; Iron 4% DV. *Recipe analyzed with almond milk, apricot fruit spread, gluten-free all purpose baking mix and without any nuts or chips.*

NUTTY CRUNCH BON BONS

I like these for their flavor and crunch. They have a nice blend of essential fatty acids and protein. They are also easy and fun to make with a child. Eating "the batter" when it sticks to your hands can create laughter and great memories for everyone involved.

⅔ cup unsalted and unsweetened hempseed butter, pumpkin seed butter or Brazil nut butter

⅔ cup unsalted and unsweetened cashew or almond butter

⅛ cup brown rice syrup or yacon syrup

⅛ tsp sea or Himalayan salt

2 tsp alcohol-free vanilla flavoring or other flavoring

1½ cup Crunchy Rice™ cereal (or Crunchy Flax™ cereal)

1. In a saucepan, combine the nut butters, sweetener and salt over very low heat. When warmed, add the flavoring and mix well.

2. Add the Crunchy Rice™ cereal and fold into the mixture.

3. With your hands (or your child's), form teaspoon-sized balls. You can also make bars by spreading the mixture evenly into the bottom of an 8 x 8 pan.

Makes: 24 bon bons or bars
Preparation time: 15 minutes
Serving size: 2 bon bons or bars

Corn-Free | *Nut and Seed-Free* | *Nut or Seed-Free* | *Soy-Free*

HINTS, TIPS AND SUBSTITUTIONS

Varying the nut or seed butters will provide different nutrients. If sensitive to nuts, use seed butter only.

Some may prefer more sweetener, depending upon taste and nut butter used.

Crunchy Rice™ *and Crunchy Flax*™ *cereals contain some honey. Gluten-free brown rice crisps work well as a substitute though may not stay as "crispy".*

Dip bon bons into chocolate sauce or drizzle sauce on top of bon bons. If you are using the pan, you can "make a picture" by drizzling the chocolate sauce onto the top of the bars. See Wendy's Wonderful Chocolate Topping *recipe on pages 163.*

For a raw version of this recipe, please see page 264.

AMOUNT PER 2 BON BON SERVING: Calories 220; Calories from Fat 120; Total Fat 14g; Saturated Fat 1g; Trans Fat 0 g; Cholesterol 0 mg; Sodium 45mg; Total Carbohydrate 17g; Dietary Fiber 2g; Sugars 3g; Protein 8g; Vitamin A 8% DV; Calcium 4% DV; Iron 15% DV. *Recipe analyzed with hempseed and unsalted almond butter, Crunchy Flax*™ *cereal and brown rice syrup. (Chocolate topping not added.)*

CHERRY CHOCO YUM BON BONS

These are full of flavor, essential fatty acids, and fiber.
They also have a pretty pinkish-purple hue.

This recipe is pictured on the cover.

½ cup chia seeds

½ cup sesame seeds

½ cup sunflower seeds (unsalted)

1 cup unweetened, unsulphured shredded organic coconut

1 cup frozen or dried cherries (if frozen, thaw and drain) or ¾ cup of
    Cherry Berry Sauce noted on page 162

1 cup golden raisins (*Mulberries are also delicious in this recipe.*)

½ cup (2 scoops) Sun Warrior Chocolate Protein®

¼ cup (1 scoop) Sun Warrior Vanilla Protein®

1 cup unsalted and unsweetened tahini

¼ plus ⅛ cup unsweetened organic canned coconut milk or coconut water

Variations:

Dates, figs, apricots, goji berries or other dried fruits may
    replace cherries or raisins. Unsulphured, unsweetened
    varieties are best.

Replace tahini with nut butters (almond, cashew, pistachio, Brazil
    nut, etc.).

Replace nuts with seeds.

1. In a Cuisinart® or blender, grind seeds, coconut, cherries, and raisins until
   ground into a moist and gooey consistency.

2. Into the food processor or blender, add the gooey mixture, ¼ cup of the chocolate protein powder and ¼ cup of the vanilla powder. Process or blend until the mixture becomes thick. Transfer this mixture into a large mixing bowl. Add the remaining amount of protein powder and mix by hand. Add tahini and coconut water, and mix until the ingredients stay together well. Add liquid stevia to suit your taste.

3. Use a teaspoon to form mixture into balls, or press mixture into an 8" pan. Chill in refrigerator or freezer.

Makes: Approx. 24 bon bons
Preparation time: 15 minutes
Serving size: 2 bon bons

Corn-Free | Nut and Seed-Free | **Nut or Seed-Free** | *Soy-Free*

Hints, Tips and Substitutions

If using Cherry Berry Sauce (see page 162), add it after grinding the seeds, coconut and raisins.

For a raw version of these bon bons, please see page 266.

Amount per 2 bon bon serving: Calories 350; Calories from Fat 210; Total Fat 24g; Saturated Fat 8g; Trans Fat 0 g; Cholesterol 0 mg; Sodium 30mg; Total Carbohydrate 21g; Dietary Fiber 4g; Sugars 12g; Protein 13g; Vitamin A 2% DV; Vitamin C 2% DV; Calcium 10% DV; Iron 30% DV. *Recipe analyzed with frozen cherries and full-fat coconut milk.*

You can also make this recipe in bar form by pressing the mixture into an 8-inch round dish before slicing.

MOLASSES "MMM" TRUFFLES

These have the distinctive taste of molasses. Vitamin C-packed camu camu and iron-rich molasses gives this tasty truffle an added boost.

1 cup unsalted, unsweetened nut and seed blend (either purchased pre-made, or prepared by hand (e.g. ½ cup almond butter plus ½ cup sunflower seed butter))

½ cup rice bran

2 tsp maca powder

2 Tbsp molasses or yacon syrup or Jerusalem artichoke syrup

1½ tsp yacon syrup

½ tsp camu camu powder

⅛ cup (1 scoop) Raw Power!™ Protein Superfood Supplement®

1 Tbsp coconut *cream* (not oil)

1 dropper lemon stevia

2 Tbsp hempseeds

3 Tbsp dried blueberries (unsweetened, corn syrup and sugar-free)

2 Tbsp dried cherries (unsweetened, corn syrup and sugar-free)

1 tsp alcohol-free vanilla flavoring

½ tsp raw cacao powder

2 dashes of cinnamon

1. Combine all ingredients in a medium bowl. Mix together with your hands or a spoon.

2. Use a teaspoon to form into truffle balls. Serve or store.

Makes: Approx. 24 truffles
Preparation time: 15 minutes
Serving size: 2 truffles

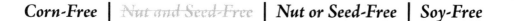

Corn-Free | ~~*Nut and Seed-Free*~~ | *Nut or Seed-Free* | *Soy-Free*

HINTS, TIPS AND SUBSTITUTIONS

If sensitive to nuts, use seed butter only.

Raw Power!™ Protein Superfood Supplement® contains nuts. Substitute a different protein powder if making a nut-free version of this recipe.

For a raw version of this recipe, please see page 268.

AMOUNT PER 2 TRUFFLE SERVING: Calories 210; Calories from Fat 120; Total Fat 13g; Saturated Fat 1.5g; Trans Fat 0g; Cholesterol 0mg; Sodium 0mg; Total Carbohydrate14g; Dietary Fiber 4g; Sugars 4g; Protein 7g; Vitamin A 2% DV; Vitamin C 2% DV; Calcium 6% DV; Iron 15% DV. *Recipe analyzed with ½ cup unsalted and unsweetened almond butter and ½ cup unsalted sunflower seed butter.*

Cakes
and Cupcakes

Many of these recipes are pictured on my
website: *www.SweetnessWithoutSugar.com*

CINNAMON SPICE BIRTHDAY CAKE (OR CUPCAKES)

Our children go to a school sanctuary called The Rose Garden, run by Sharifa Oppenheimer. This "veganized" version of "The Rose Garden" cake is light, fluffy, and delicious; it also serves as a nice brunch coffee cake. A treat to be enjoyed with friends. Sharifa has written a wonderful book for families. Please see the Appendix and Resources section on page 316.

1½ cup quinoa flour, ¼ cup arrowroot powder, ½ cup gluten-free oat flour, ¾ cup millet flour

1½ Tbsp aluminum-free baking powder

½ tsp sea or Himalayan salt

¾ tsp xanthan gum (or use guar gum if corn-sensitive)

2 or more tsp cinnamon

2 Tbsp ground flax seed (ground in coffee grinder) plus ¼ cup warm filtered water

1 tsp ground chia seeds (ground in coffee grinder) plus ⅛ cup warm filtered water

½ cup organic unrefined walnut or sunflower oil

½ cup unsweetened rice milk

½ cup unsweetened hemp milk

1½ tsp alcohol-free vanilla flavoring

¾ cup brown rice syrup or pure maple syrup (unprocessed without added corn syrup or sweetener)

1. Preheat oven to 350°F. Grease one or two 8- or 9-inch round cake pans.

2. In a large bowl, mix together flours, baking powder, salt, xanthan gum and cinnamon. Set aside.

3. In a small bowl or measuring cup, combine ground flax seed with water and set aside. In a separate small bowl, combine ground chia seeds with water and set aside. In a large bowl, mix together oil, milks, vanilla and syrup. Then add the flax/water and chia/water mixtures to the large bowl.

4. Add the wet ingredients to the dry ones. Whisk ingredients together until the batter is creamy and smooth. If you have children, invite them to help mix for you! Be careful not to overmix.

5. Pour into round cake pan or, if making two cakes, pour equal amounts into the two pans.

6. Bake for 20-25 minutes (Baking time may be longer with different sweeteners; start at 20 minutes and test). Cake is done when lightly browned on top and when a tester placed in the center of the cake (or cupcake) comes out clean.

7. Let the cake cool completely. This cake is delicate, so use extra care when removing it from the pan. For best results, refrigerate the layers before frosting.

Makes: 32 single-layer slices; 2 (8-9-inch) cake pans;
Approx. 24 cupcakes/muffins (filled ½ with batter)
Preparation time: 20-25 minutes
Baking time: cake 20-25 mins. / cupcakes/muffins 15-20 mins.
Serving size: 1 slice cake or 2 cupcakes/muffins

Corn-Free* | ~~Nut and Seed-Free~~ | **Nut or Seed-Free** | **Soy-Free**

* Check labels

HINTS, TIPS AND SUBSTITUTIONS

If you are sensitive to nuts or seeds, use only rice milk. Consistency of cake may differ with different milks.

This recipe also works well as a "vamilla" cupcake.

For a taller, traditional-sized cake, pour all of the ingredients into one 8- or 9-inch round pan (rather than two).

AMOUNT PER 1 SLICE CAKE OF 32 OR 2 CUPCAKES SERVING: Calories 220; Calories from Fat 80; Total Fat 9g; Saturated Fat 1g Trans Fat 0g; Cholesterol 0mg; Sodium 230mg; Total Carbohydrate 31g; Dietary Fiber 3g; Sugars 9g; Protein 3g; Calcium 6% DV; Iron 8% DV. *Recipe analyzed with sunflower oil and brown rice syrup.*

YUMMY TUMMY CHOCOLATE CAKE (OR CUPCAKES)

This recipe was originally inspired from Sarah Kramer and Tanya Barnard's <u>How It All Vegan!</u> at www.govegan.net and was printed with their permission in the first edition of <u>Sweetness Without Sugar</u>. This revised version offers a delicious combination for those who love moist, "chocolaty" cupcakes with a molasses taste. If you prefer a more traditional chocolate cupcake without a molasses taste, make these with brown rice syrup, pure maple syrup or yacon syrup. These cupcakes even contain iron and protein.

1 cup blackstrap molasses or ½ cup yacon or ½ cup brown rice syrup or
    ½ cup pure maple syrup (unprocessed without added corn syrup
    or sweetener)

1 cup unsweetened hemp milk

2 cups fruit-sweetened, allergen- and dairy-free chocolate chips
    (one 10-oz. bag) or 1½ cups vegan carob chips
    (*These chips may contain cane sugar.*)

2 tsp ground chia seeds (ground in coffee grinder) plus ¼ cup warm
    filtered water

¼ cup organic unrefined walnut or sunflower oil

1 tsp alcohol-free vanilla flavoring

4 Tbsp dried arrowroot powder

1¾ cups gluten-free all-purpose baking mix

¼ cup gluten-free oat flour

¾ tsp xanthan gum (or use guar gum if corn-sensitive)

1. Preheat oven to 375°F. Lightly grease the cake or muffin pan with unrefined oil.

2. In a saucepan, whisk together the sweetener, ½ cup milk and the chips. Cook over low heat, until the chips have melted. Stir constantly.

3. In a separate bowl, combine the chia seeds and water and set aside. Add oil, vanilla, and arrowroot to the melted and warmed chocolate mixture. Remove from heat, add the chia/water mixture and set aside.

4. In a different bowl, combine the flours, xanthan gum and the rest of the milk. Then add the chocolate mixture and stir with a spoon until thoroughly mixed. *If the flours clump together, use a handmixer to create a smooth batter.*

5. Spoon into a lightly greased cupcake pan or into liners and bake for 15 minutes. Check for doneness (with a toothpick inserted in the middle) and if necessary, bake for an additional 5 minutes. This batter can also be poured into a 9-inch round cake pan.

Makes: 16 slices; 1 (8-9 inch) cake;
Approx. 20 cupcakes/muffins (filled ½ with batter)
Preparation time: 30 minutes
Baking time: cake 15 - 30 mins. / cupcakes/muffins 10 - 15 mins.
Serving size: 1 slice cake or 1 cupcake/muffin

Corn-Free* | ~~Nut and Seed-Free~~ | **Nut or Seed-Free** | *Soy-Free*

* Check labels

HINTS, TIPS AND SUBSTITUTIONS

For a more "traditional" chocolate cupcake, replace molasses with either brown rice syrup, pure maple syrup or yacon syrup. You may prefer to use less alternative sweetener, depending upon your taste.

Can substitute rice milk for the hemp milk if you are sensitive to seeds.

Packaged carob chips may contain gluten and corn. To make your own carob chips, see page 184 for a stevia-sweetened option.

Some gluten-free flours containing high amounts of rice, potato, arrowroot, cornstarch and other higher-glycemic grains may raise blood sugar more than bean-based gluten-free flours. If you are a diabetic, please check your blood sugar after eating this treat. Experiment with different sweeteners and sweetener quantities to determine what combination works best for you.

You can use a mini muffin pan for a smaller portion size. Mini muffins are very sweet and work well for a special "pop in your mouth" lunch box treat. This recipe makes 1 tray of 24 mini muffins plus a small heart-shaped cake.

AMOUNT PER 1 SLICE CAKE OF 16 OR 1 CUPCAKE SERVING: Calories 220; Calories from Fat 100; Total Fat 11g; Saturated Fat 4.5g; Trans Fat 0g; Cholesterol 0mg; Sodium 130mg; Total Carbohydrate 31g; Dietary Fiber 2g; Sugars 13g; Protein 3g; Iron 2% DV *Recipe analyzed with brown rice syrup, dairy-free chips containing cane juice and unsweetened hemp milk.*

COMFORT FOOD CARROT CAKE (OR CUPCAKES)

This recipe was originally inspired from Sarah Kramer and Tanya Barnard's <u>How It All Vegan!</u> at www.govegan.net and was printed with their permission in the first edition of <u>Sweetness Without Sugar</u>. This revised version is easy to make and is delicious as a birthday cake or a protein-filled breakfast treat. With this recipe, even "picky eaters" will enjoy eating their vegetables!

1¼ cup gluten-free flour or baking mix

¼ cup gluten-free oat flour

¼ cup (1 scoop) Sun Warrior Natural Protein[R] (optional)

½ cup maple or coconut sugar crystals (or less to suit your taste)

2 tsp baking powder (*Omit if using a flour mix containing baking powder.*)

½ tsp xanthan gum (or use guar gum if corn-sensitive)

1 tsp cinnamon

¼ tsp sea or Himalayan salt

1 tsp ground chia seeds (ground in coffee grinder) plus ⅛ cup warm filtered water

1 Tbsp ground flax seed (ground in coffee grinder) plus ⅛ cup warm filtered water

¾ cup hemp or almond milk (unsweetened and either vanilla or unflavored)

2 tsp alcohol-free vanilla flavoring

¼ cup organic unrefined walnut or sunflower oil

¾ cup carrot, finely shredded (by hand or with food processor) (about 1½ carrots)

1 tsp fresh ginger, grated (or ground in a coffee grinder)

1. Preheat oven to 350°F. Lightly grease an 8- or 9-inch pie pan with unrefined oil.

2. In a large bowl, stir together the flours, protein powder (if using), sweetener, baking powder, xanthan gum, cinnamon, and salt. In a separate bowl or measuring cup, combine the chia seeds and water. Do the same with the flax/water mixture. Set both of these seed mixtures aside. In another large bowl, add the dairy-free milk, vanilla, oil, chia and flax seed mixtures, carrot and ginger, and lightly mix together.

3. Combine the wet and dry ingredients and stir briefly with a spoon until a thick batter is formed.

4. Pour into a lightly oiled 8 x 8 pan or 8- or 9-inch round cake pan and bake for 25-30 minutes. With a knife or toothpick, check for doneness. Cake may not rise as high as a conventional cake. After the cake has cooled, enjoy a plain slice, or top with *To-Tootin Fruit-In Topping* on page 159 and serve. This recipe also makes delicious muffins.

Makes: 16 square pieces or 8 slices cake,
12 muffins (filled ½ with batter)
Preparation time: 25 minutes
Baking time: cake 25-30 mins. / cupcakes/muffins 20-25 mins.
Serving size: 1 slice cake or 1-2 cupcakes/muffins

Corn-Free* | ~~Nut and Seed-Free~~ | **Nut or Seed-Free** | *Soy-Free*

* Check labels

HINTS, TIPS AND SUBSTITUTIONS

Gluten-free baking mixes often contain baking powder. If this is the case with your flour, please omit the baking powder. When using the Arrowhead Mills All Purpose Baking Flour®, you will want to add the baking powder anyway to achieve a moist consistency.

For a taller, traditional-sized cake, double the recipe and pour into an 8- or 9-inch round pan.

AMOUNT PER 1 SLICE CAKE OF 8 SERVINGS IN A ROUND CAKE PAN OR A 2 PIECE SERVING (IN A SQUARE PAN): Calories 200; Calories from Fat 80; Total Fat 9g; Saturated Fat 1g Trans Fat 0g; Cholesterol 0mg; Sodium 400mg; Total Carbohydrate 28g; Dietary Fiber 2g; Sugars 5g; Protein 4g; Vitamin A 35% DV; Vitamin C 2% DV; Calcium 6% DV; Iron 4% DV *Recipe analyzed with Hemp Bliss*[R] *unsweetened hemp milk, ½ cup maple sugar crystals and sunflower oil.*

AMOUNT PER 1 SLICE CAKE OF 8 SERVINGS IN A ROUND CAKE PAN OR A 2 PIECE SERVING (IN A SQUARE PAN) WITH SUN WARRIOR® ADDED: Calories 210; Calories from Fat 80; Total Fat 9g; Saturated Fat 1g Trans Fat 0g; Cholesterol 0mg; Sodium 370mg; Total Carbohydrate 28g; Dietary Fiber 2g; Sugars 5g; Protein 6g; Vitamin A 35% DV; Vitamin C 2% DV; Calcium 15% DV; Iron 6% DV *Recipe analyzed with Sun Warrior protein*[R]*, Hemp Bliss*[R] *unsweetened hemp milk, ½ cup maple sugar crystals and sunflower oil.*

AMOUNT PER 1 CUPCAKE WITH SUN WARRIOR PROTEIN[R] **ADDED:** Calories 140; Calories from Fat 50; Total Fat 6g; Saturated Fat .5g Trans Fat 0g; Cholesterol 0mg; Sodium 250mg; Total Carbohydrate 19g; Dietary Fiber 1g; Sugars 3g; Protein 4g; Vitamin A 25% DV; Calcium 8% DV; Iron 4% DV *Recipe analyzed with Sun Warrior protein*[R]*, Hemp Bliss*[R] *unsweetened hemp milk, ½ cup maple sugar crystals and sunflower oil. Muffin cups filled half-way with raw batter.*

AMOUNT PER 1 CUPCAKE WITHOUT PROTEIN POWDER: Calories 130; Calories from Fat 50; Total Fat 6g; Saturated Fat .5g Trans Fat 0g; Cholesterol 0mg; Sodium 240mg; Total Carbohydrate 19g; Dietary Fiber 1g; Sugars 3g; Protein 3g; Vitamin A 25% DV; Calcium 8% DV; Iron 2% DV *Recipe analyzed with Hemp Bliss*[R] *unsweetened hemp milk, ½ cup maple sugar crystals and sunflower oil. Muffin cups filled half-way with raw batter.*

TO-TOOTIN' FRUIT-IN TOPPING

Recipe adapted from Sarah Kramer and Tanya Barnard's _How It All Vegan!_ Printed with permission from _How It All Vegan!_ www.govegan.net

This tasty topping is easy to make and goes nicely with Comfort Food Carrot Cake and other sweet goodies.

1 cup soft or medium tofu (packaged in water)

¼ cup cashew pieces or macadamia nuts

4 tsp brown rice syrup or yacon syrup (or adjust amounts to suit your taste)

½ tsp sea or Himalayan salt

½ cup fruit (strawberries, blueberries, etc.)

1. In a blender or food processor, blend together all the ingredients until smooth and thick.

2. Spread on cakes, cupcakes or other sweet treats. _This topping spreads best when refrigerated for four hours or more._

3. Store in a sealable container. Will keep in refrigerator 4-7 days.

Makes: 2 cups
Preparation time: 10 minutes
Serving size: ⅛ cup or 2 Tbsp

Corn-Free | Nut and Seed-Free | **Nut or Seed-Free** | Soy-Free

AMOUNT PER ⅛ CUP OR 2 TBSP SERVING: Calories 40; Calories from Fat 20; Total Fat 2g; Saturated Fat 0g; Trans Fat 0g; Cholesterol 0mg; Sodium 45mg; Total Carbohydrate 3g; Dietary Fiber 0g; Sugars 1g; Protein 2g; Vitamin C 4% DV; Calcium 2% DV; Iron 2% DV. _Recipe analyzed with brown rice syrup, cashews and strawberries._

EASY CREAM CHEESE FROSTING

1 container Tofutti® Better Than Cream Cheese, plain

¼ cup brown rice syrup or liquid stevia to taste

Filtered water to desired consistency

1. Combine ingredients and blend well in blender or with a hand mixer. Add filtered water until you achieve your desired consistency, until smooth and spreadable.

2. Spread frosting on your favorite desserts and cakes.

Makes: Approx. 1 cup

Preparation time: 10 minutes

Serving size: ⅛ cup or 2 Tbsp

Corn-Free* | *Nut and Seed-Free* | *Nut or Seed-Free* | *Soy-Free*

* Check labels

HINTS, TIPS AND SUBSTITUTIONS

Tofutti® contains soy isolates, hydrogenated soybean oil and sugar in several forms. Look for the non-hydrogenated version (a yellow container). I include this recipe as a quick vegan frosting idea.

AMOUNT PER ⅛ CUP OR 2 TBSP SERVING: Calories 120; Calories from Fat 80; Total Fat 9g; Saturated Fat 2g; Trans Fat 0g; Cholesterol 0mg; Sodium 160mg; Total Carbohydrate 10g; Dietary Fiber 0g; Sugars 6g; Protein 1g. *Recipe analyzed with brown rice syrup; stevia can be added for extra sweetness.*

BASIC BUTTERCREAM TOPPING

This vegan "butter"-cream frosting makes vegan desserts even more delicious. It's perfect for vegan treats you bring to potlucks or parties where the majority of guests are non-vegan and might like to enjoy what you bring.

1 lb silken organic firm tofu, drained (12-oz. box, non-refrigerated, also works well)

3½ Tbsp brown rice syrup or yacon syrup

6 Tbsp xylitol (ground in coffee grinder)

4½ tsp alcohol-free vanilla flavoring

1¼ cup organic (non-GMO) Earth Balance® spread

1-2 Tbsp lemon juice (optional) (*If using store-bought lemon juice, less juice may be required to suit your taste.*)

1. Combine all ingredients. Using a blender or hand mixer, mix ingredients thoroughly, until smooth and spreadable. If you prefer a colored topping, use natural decorating colors (*see the* Appendix and Resources *section on page 302*).

2. Add to your favorite desserts and cakes. *This topping spreads best when refrigerated for four hours or more.*

Makes: Approx. 3 cups

Preparation time: 10 minutes

Serving size: 1 piece of single layer cake, topped (about 2 Tbsp topping)

Corn-Free* | Nut and Seed-Free | Nut or Seed-Free | Soy-Free

* Check labels

HINTS, TIPS AND SUBSTITUTIONS

This topping will cover one round two-layer cake (8" or 9" rounds). It tastes delicious with the Yummy Tummy Chocolate Cake *on page 154 and/or the* Comfort Food Carrot Cake *on page 156.*

AMOUNT PER ⅛ CUP OR 2 Tbsp serving: Calories 110; Calories from Fat 90; Total Fat 10g; Saturated Fat 3g; Trans Fat 0g; Cholesterol 0mg; Sodium 105mg; Total Carbohydrate 6g; Dietary Fiber 0g; Sugars 2g; Protein 1g; Vitamin A 8% DV; Calcium 2% DV. *Recipe analyzed with brown rice syrup and 1 Tbsp lemon juice.*

CHERRY BERRY SAUCE

This is a nice sauce to pour over brownies,
"ice creams", cereal, smoothies and more.

2 cups unsweetened frozen cherries (*Can use cranberries in season,*
during holiday time.)

¼ cup xylitol or maple or coconut sugar crystals

½ cup filtered water (*Use less for a thicker consistency.*)

½ tsp alcohol-free almond flavoring (*Those with nut allergies may select a*
different flavoring.)

1. In a small saucepan, over medium-high heat, combine cherries, sweetener, water and flavoring.

2. Cover and simmer until the cherries soften and juices form, stirring occasionally, about 8 minutes.

3. Cool cherry mixture slightly and then pureé in blender until smooth. Drizzle over brownies, "ice cream", frozen yogurt, smoothies, cookies, cereal, pancakes and more. *Can also use this sauce in the* Cherry Choco Yum Bon Bons *on page 146.* Store remainder in the refrigerator.

Makes: 1½ cups
Preparation time: 10 minutes
Serving size: ¼ cup

Corn-Free | *Nut and Seed-Free* | *Nut or Seed-Free* | *Soy-Free*

AMOUNT PER ¼ CUP SERVING: Calories 45; Calories from Fat 0; Total Fat 0g; Saturated Fat 0g; Trans Fat 0g; Cholesterol 0mg; Sodium 0mg; Total Carbohydrate 15g; Dietary Fiber 1g; Sugars 5g; Protein 0g; Vitamin A 8% DV ;Vitamin C 2% DV; Iron 2% DV. *Recipe analyzed with unsweetened frozen cherries and xylitol.*

WENDY'S WONDERFUL CHOCOLATE TOPPING

If you are a chocolate lover, it is hard to create a bad chocolate sauce. I recommend using a high-quality cocoa that is at least 70% cacao. Truth be told, even if a dessert doesn't taste as good as you had hoped, adding a little bit of one of these toppings "makes it all better." This and the toppings on the following pages have some slight variations between them and they are all delicious! Enjoy!

½ cup fruit-sweetened, allergen- and dairy-free chocolate chips or 1½

cups vegan carob chips (*These chips may contain cane sugar.*)

½ cup unsweetened organic canned coconut milk or unsweetened,

dairy-free milk (e.g. almond, brown rice or hemp milk)

1. In a saucepan, melt chocolate with the coconut milk or dairy-free milk, until smooth.

2. Drizzle over your favorite dessert.

Makes: 1 cup
Preparation time: 10 minutes
Serving size: ⅛ cup or 2 Tbsp

Corn-Free* | Nut and Seed-Free | Nut or Seed-Free | Soy-Free

* Check labels

HINTS, TIPS AND SUBSTITUTIONS

Packaged carob chips may contain gluten and corn. To make your own carob chips, see page 184 for a stevia-sweetened option.

This topping tastes spectacular with the Coconut Macaroons noted on page 192.

AMOUNT PER ⅛ CUP OR 2 TBSP SERVING: Calories 80; Calories from Fat 60; Total Fat 7g; Saturated Fat 5g Trans Fat 0g; Cholesterol 0 mg; Sodium 0mg; Total Carbohydrate 7g; Dietary Fiber 1g; Sugars 6g; Protein 1g; Iron 2% DV. *Recipe analyzed with pure, unsweetened, regular-fat coconut milk.*

VANILLA CHOCOLATE SAUCE

This recipe was inspired by Ann Gentry's recipe for chocolate sauce in <u>The Real Food Daily Cookbook</u>. This sauce tastes fabulous on the Coconut and Creamy Pie (on page 220), and with many other desserts presented in this book. The ingredients combine well, creating a sauce that can be made as thick or thin as you like.

¾ cup unsweetened, dairy-free cocoa powder

¼ -½ cup pure maple syrup (unprocessed without added corn syrup or sweetener) (*Brown rice syrup, yacon syrup or liquid stevia can replace maple syrup.*)

1½ tsp alcohol-free vanilla flavoring

2 tablespoons unsweetened, dairy-free milk (e.g. almond, brown rice or hemp milk)

1. In a bowl, combine the cocoa powder, sweetener and the vanilla. Whisk in enough of the dairy-free milk to form a thin sauce. *If using stevia, more dairy-free milk will be needed to create the desired consistency.*

2. Drizzle over your favorite dessert.

Makes: Approx. 1¼ cups
Preparation time: 10 minutes
Serving size: ⅛ cup or 2 Tbsp

Corn-Free* | Nut and Seed-Free | Nut or Seed-Free | Soy-Free

* Check labels

HINTS, TIPS AND SUBSTITUTIONS

See the Appendix and Resources *section on page 306 for dairy-free cocoa and milk suggestions.*

See chart on page 104 to determine the amount of stevia to use in this recipe.

AMOUNT PER ⅛ CUP OR 2 TBSP SERVING: Calories 70; Calories from Fat 10; Total Fat 1.5g; Saturated Fat 0g Trans Fat 0g; Cholesterol 0mg; Sodium 0mg; Total Carbohydrate 14g; Dietary Fiber 2g; Sugars 11g; Protein 1g; Iron 6% DV. *Recipe analyzed with ½ cup pure maple syrup and unsweetened hemp milk. Using less pure maple syrup or one of the other sweeteners listed will provide less sugar per serving.*

CHA CHA FOR CHOCOLATE TOPPING

1½ cups fruit-sweetened, allergen- and dairy-free chocolate chips or 1½
cups vegan carob chips (*These chips may contain cane sugar.*)

⅔ cup unsweetened, dairy-free milk (e.g. almond, brown rice or hemp milk),
plain variety

Liquid stevia to taste

1. In a saucepan, melt chocolate with dairy-free milk, until smooth.

2. Drizzle over your favorite dessert and enjoy.

Makes: ¾ cup
Preparation time: 10 minutes
Serving size: ⅛ cup or 2 Tbsp

Corn-Free* | Nut and Seed-Free | Nut or Seed-Free | Soy-Free

* Check labels

HINTS, TIPS AND SUBSTITUTIONS

*Packaged carob chips may contain gluten and corn. To make your
own carob chips, see page 184 for a stevia-sweetened option.*

AMOUNT PER ⅛ CUP OR 2 TBSP SERVING: Calories 240; Calories from Fat
140; Total Fat 16g; Saturated Fat 9g Trans Fat 0g; Cholesterol 0mg; Sodium
0mg; Total Carbohydrate 27g; Dietary Fiber 3g; Sugars 21g; Protein 4g. *Recipe
analyzed with chocolate chips (with cane sugar) and unsweetened hemp milk.*

LOCO FOR CHOCO SAUCE

½ cup unsweetened, dairy-free cocoa powder

¼ cup either unsweetened organic canned coconut milk or coconut
water or unsweetened, dairy-free milk. (*Begin with ¼ cup liquid.
If desired, add more liquid to create a thinner consistency.*)

5 drops liquid stevia, plain or flavored (*Add more drops to suit your taste.*)

1. In a saucepan, melt chocolate with the liquid, until smooth. While mixing, add enough stevia to suit your taste.

2. Drizzle over your favorite dessert and enjoy.

Makes: Approx. ¾ cup (variable depending on liquid used)
Preparation time: 10 minutes
Serving size: ⅛ cup or 2 Tbsp

Corn-Free* | *Nut and Seed-Free* | *Nut or Seed-Free* | *Soy-Free*

* Check labels

HINTS, TIPS AND SUBSTITUTIONS

See the Appendix and Resources *section on page 306 for dairy-free cocoa suggestions*

For a raw version of this recipe, please see page 270.

AMOUNT PER ⅛ CUP OR 2 TBSP SERVING: Calories 35; Calories from Fat 15; Total Fat 1.5g; Saturated Fat 0g Trans Fat 0g; Cholesterol 0mg; Sodium 40mg; Total Carbohydrate 6g; Dietary Fiber 3g; Sugars 1g; Protein 2g; Iron 6% DV; Vitamin C 2% DV. *Recipe analyzed with 1 cup of the 10 oz. can of Edward & Son's coconut water.*

Cookies

and Bars

Many of these recipes are pictured on my
website: *www.SweetnessWithoutSugar.com*

NUTTER NUMMY SQUARES

Delicious and decadent and almost effortless. I remember eating Nabisco Nutter Butter® cookies as a child. They were shaped in a square with a crispy outside and delicious peanut butter inside. These squares have the two textures minus corn syrup, artificial ingredients, GMO's and hydrogenated fats. Delightfully satisfying.

CRUST BOTTOM:
Select a crust recipe on pages 212-217.

NUTTY FILLING:
¾ cup unsweetened and unsalted almond, cashew, hempseed or Brazil
  nut butter

¼ cup ground xylitol (*Can substitute with ground maple or
  coconut sugar crystals.*)

½ tsp sea or Himalayan salt

⅜ cup unsweetened, dairy-free milk (e.g. almond, brown rice or hemp milk),
  plain variety

½ tsp alcohol-free vanilla flavoring (optional)

CHOCOLATE TOPPING:
Choose from toppings on pages 163-166.

1. In a saucepan over medium-high heat, combine nut butter, sweetener, salt, and dairy-free milk. Stir until mixed together. When this mixture begins to thicken, add vanilla and remove from heat. Continue to stir until mixture is thick but pourable. Do not boil.

2. Pour mixture over your chosen baked crust in an 8 x 8 pan. *Use the amount of crust for your desired thickness. If you prefer to taste more "nutty num" than crust, use less of the crust on the bottom of the pan. The "nutty num" mixture forms about ½ to ¾ inch thickness once poured, cooled and firm.*

3. Chill bars in refrigerator for 30 minutes to 1 hour. While the bars cool, prepare a chocolate topping (if desired) noted on pages 163-166.

4. Top with chocolate topping and re-chill until ready to eat (if you can wait that long).

Makes: 16 bars
Preparation and baking time: 25 minutes
Chill and cool time: 30 minutes to 1 hour
Serving size: 1 bar

Corn-Free* | ~~Nut and Seed-Free~~ | **Nut or Seed-Free** | *Soy-Free*

* Check labels

HINTS, TIPS AND SUBSTITUTIONS

Different nut butters and nut butter brands have different consistencies when heated or refrigerated. If your filling is "runnier" than desired, use a little more nut butter. Adding about 1 teaspoon or less of arrowroot starch will also help thicken the nut mixture upon heating.

To balance the sweet and salty flavors present in the topping and crust, you may prefer to add less than ¾ tsp salt to the filling.

Adding vanilla to this recipe will make the topping slightly brown. This will occur when using either vanilla flavoring or dairy-free unsweetened milk containing vanilla.

See page 218 for the recipe for Nutter Nummy Pie.

AMOUNT PER 1 SQUARE OF 16 SERVING: Calories 220; Calories from Fat 130; Total Fat 14g; Saturated Fat 1g; Trans Fat 0g; Cholesterol 0mg; Sodium 125mg; Total Carbohydrate 19g; Dietary Fiber 3g; Sugars 3g; Protein 6g; Calcium 6% DV; Iron 6% DV *Recipe analyzed with almond butter, xylitol, and unsweetened hemp milk for the filling, the Loco for Choco Sauce on page 166 and Wendy's Pie Crust with Nuts on page 214.*

FUDGE

This recipe was inspired by other delicious raw fudge recipes. It can be prepared with carob or chocolate. Many people have asked for this recipe and are amazed that the sweet taste comes only from fruits and the hint of coconut oil.

¾ cup unrefined, virgin coconut oil, warmed until liquid (measure ¾ cup of melted oil)

1 cup pitted soft dates

½ cup mulberries, raisins, currants, dried cherries or goji berries

1 tsp maca (optional; adds more superfood nutrition)

Dash of cinnamon

1 tsp alcohol-free vanilla flavoring

¼ cup carob powder

¼ cup unsweetened, dairy-free cocoa powder or cacao

¼ cup extra carob or unsweetened, dairy-free cocoa powder or cacao

⅓ cup (about 2 scoops) Sun Warrior Protein® or (about 4 scoops) Raw Power!™ Protein Superfood Supplement

1½ cups walnuts, soaked 2 hours, then drained and dried (still yummy without these too)

1. In a small saucepan, melt the coconut oil and measure to ¾ cup. Use a food processor to blend the dates, berries of choice and coconut oil. Process until smooth.

2. Add maca (if using), cinnamon, vanilla, raw chocolate (or carob), and protein powder and process again.

3. Transfer the mixture from a food processor into a bowl and add the walnuts (if using).

4. Knead the walnuts into the mixture. Pack the fudge firmly into an 8 x 8 pan. Fudge should be approximately one-inch thick. Slice into 16 pieces.

5. Refrigerate for an hour prior to serving. Fudge stored in a closed container in the refrigerator will last up to one month.

Makes: 16 pieces
Preparation time: 25 minutes
Serving size: 1 piece

Corn-Free* | *Nut and Seed-Free* | *Nut or Seed-Free* | *Soy-Free*

* Check labels

Hints, Tips and Substitutions

Preparing this fudge in steps, as noted above, makes a difference since it is a thick mixture. Though I often just put things together and blend, for this recipe, I recommend following the instructions.

This recipe can be prepared by replacing the ¼ cup carob, ¼ cup carob or cacao, and ¼ cup carob, cacao or cocoa, with 1) ¾ cup carob only, or 2) ¾ cup dairy-free cocoa only.

See the Appendix and Resources *section on page 306 for dairy-free cocoa and superfood suggestions (see pages 312-314).*

For a raw version of this recipe, please see page 272.

Amount per 1 piece serving: Calories 220; Calories from Fat 130; Total Fat 15g; Saturated Fat 7g; Trans Fat 0g; Cholesterol 0mg; Sodium 10mg; Total Carbohydrate 16g; Dietary Fiber 2g; Sugars 15g; Protein 6g; Vitamin C 15% DV; Calcium 4% DV; Iron 6% DV *Recipe analyzed with mulberries, ¾ cup raw cacao, Sun Warrior Protein® and walnuts.*

The fruits and superfoods in this fudge contain beneficial nutrients. The fudge is also made with cacao/chocolate, which affects people differently. My recommendation is to listen to your body when determining your optimum serving size.

RICE CRISPY TREATS

I have fond memories of eating Rice Krispies Treats™. Inspired by various recipes (including Cynthia Lair's), these treats are definitely kid and adult approved! I've offered them at classes, potlucks and other gatherings, receiving excellent feedback from people of all ages. These treats are fondly referred to in our house as "cripsies," by our kids. Although sweet, they contain healthy fats and some protein to help balance blood sugar and bring smiles to all.

2 tsp unrefined, virgin coconut oil or organic, GMO-free Earth Balance®

1 cup brown rice syrup

5 Tbsp unsalted and unsweetened almond butter (*Can also use other nut or seed butters.*)

2-3 Tbsp unrefined coconut *cream* (not oil)

2 tsp alcohol-free vanilla (or other) flavoring

6 cups dry, natural, gluten-free, brown rice crispy cereal (e.g. approx. 1 box)

1. Set out all ingredients before beginning, because preparation goes fast!

2. Melt oil in a large pot on medium heat. Stir in rice syrup, nut butter and cream. When the bubbles form, turn off the heat.

3. Optional: Though these treats are yummy without extras, feel free to add fruit-sweetened, allergen- and dairy-free chocolate chips or vegan carob chips. (*These chips may contain cane sugar.*) If you want to add other ingredients, consider raisins, goji berries or other dried fruit. If using one of these additional ingredients, begin with one at a time (measured at ¼ to ½ cup total) to keep the texture of the treats chewy and soft.

4. Add vanilla and cereal to the pot. Mix thoroughly.

5. With a spoon, spread mixture into a 13 x 9 inch pan. Moisten your hands and press the rest down until it spreads evenly in the pan.

6. Allow the treats to cool before slicing. *For extra fun, cut the treats into shapes and sprinkle each with a dash of spirulina powder to make trees or tree people. For gooey, sticky and soft treats, store them in an airtight container.*

Makes: 24 bars
Preparation and cooking time: 10 minutes
Serving size: 1-2 bars

Corn-Free* | ~~*Nut and Seed-Free*~~ | *Nut or Seed-Free* | *Soy-Free*

* Check labels

HINTS, TIPS AND SUBSTITUTIONS

If you are sensitive to soy, use the soy-free (red container) version of Earth Balance®.

Using less sweetener (¾ cup) results in a delicious end product that is less gooey.

If you are sensitive to nuts and seeds but tolerate soy, use an organic, GMO-free soy butter.

Packaged carob chips may contain gluten and corn. To make your own carob chips, see page 184 for a stevia-sweetened option.

AMOUNT PER 1 BAR SERVING: Calories 110; Calories from Fat 30; Total Fat 3g; Saturated Fat 1g; Trans Fat 0g; Cholesterol 0mg; Sodium 25mg; Total Carbohydrate 20g; Dietary Fiber 1g; Sugars 8g; Protein 2g; Calcium 2% DV; Iron 2% DV. *Recipe analyzed with coconut oil, 1 cup brown rice syrup, almond butter and 2 ½ Tbsp coconut cream.*

OATMEAL GOJI COOKIES

The goji berries give these cookies a nice, unique flavor. I originally prepared these for a holiday treat, adding hemp protein to make a "green and red" cookie. Both protein choices work well. If the "green" color is unfavorable in your home, use the Sun Warrior Protein® instead.

1½ cups rolled oats (use certified gluten-free oats)

1 cup brown rice flour or millet flour

⅓ cup organic hemp protein powder or Sun Warrior Protein®

¾ tsp xanthan gum (or use guar gum if corn-sensitive)

¼ tsp sea or Himalayan salt

4 Tbsp ground flax seed (ground in coffee grinder) plus ⅜ cup warm
    filtered water

½ cup yacon syrup or brown rice syrup or pure maple syrup
    (unprocessed without added corn syrup or sweetener) (*Use up to
    ¾ cup sweetener to suit your taste.*)

¾ cup walnut or sunflower or unrefined, virgin coconut oil (*If using
    coconut oil, measure ¾ cup after melting.*)

½ tsp cinnamon

1 tsp alcohol-free vanilla flavoring

⅓ cup goji berries

1. Preheat oven to 350°F. Lightly grease two cookie sheets with unrefined, virgin coconut oil.

2. Combine oats, flour, protein powder, xanthan gum and salt. Set aside.

3. In a small bowl or measuring cup, combine ground flax seed with water and set aside. In another bowl mix together sweetener, oil, cinnamon, vanilla and goji berries. Combine the two wet mixtures in one bowl.

4. Add wet ingredients to dry mixture and mix well.

5. Using a tablespoon, drop cookies onto a lightly oiled cookie sheet.

6. Bake 15 minutes or until lightly browned.

Makes: 26 cookies
Preparation time: 15 minutes
Baking time: 15 minutes
Serving size: 2 cookies

Corn-Free | ~~*Nut and Seed-Free*~~ | *Nut or Seed-Free* | *Soy-Free*

HINTS, TIPS AND SUBSTITUTIONS

You may also substitute quinoa flakes for oats. To make a "prettier" version, grind the oats and/or quinoa flakes for a more uniform cookie.

The small amount of sweetener makes these an excellent treat to carry with you for snacks, and "to go" nourishment.

AMOUNT PER 2 COOKIE SERVING: Calories 260; Calories from Fat 130; Total Fat 15g; Saturated Fat 2g; Trans Fat 0g; Cholesterol 0mg; Sodium 60mg; Total Carbohydrate 27g; Dietary Fiber 4g; Sugars 9g; Protein 5g; Calcium 2% DV; Iron 10% DV. *Recipe analyzed with ½ cup brown rice syrup, hemp protein and walnut oil.*

If you like a cookie that is moist and chewy, add ¼ cup (or more) oil, or one extra tablespoon of flax seed plus another ⅛ cup warm filtered water. This will give the cookies a hearty, "stick to your ribs" texture.

"BREADY" BANANA BROWNIES

These were inspired by my husband's Aunt Ellie's banana bread. We have memories of eating it together over the holidays. My sister also made this healthy, sweet bread for us to enjoy after our son Solomon was born.

2 cups brown rice flour

1½ cups almond or hazelnut meal/flour

4½ tsp aluminum-free baking powder

½ tsp baking soda

½ tsp xanthan gum (or use guar gum if corn-sensitive)

⅔ cup or less maple or coconut sugar crystals (ground in coffee grinder)

4 Tbsp ground flax seed (ground in coffee grinder) plus ½ cup warm filtered water

4 ripe bananas, mashed

⅔ cup organic unrefined walnut or sunflower oil

½ cup fruit-sweetened, allergen- and dairy-free chocolate chips or ½ cup

      vegan carob chips (*These chips may contain cane sugar.*)

1. Preheat oven to 350°F. Lightly grease an 8 x 8 pan with unrefined, virgin coconut oil. *This recipe also works well in a loaf pan, muffin pan or an 8-inch round cake pan.*

2. In a bowl, combine the flours, baking powder, baking soda, xanthan gum and ground sweetener. Lightly mix these ingredients together.

3. In a separate dish, combine the flax seed with water and set aside. In a separate bowl, mash the bananas, add the oil and then the flax-water mixture. Stir into the dry ingredients. Add chocolate chips (if using) and fold them into the mixture.

4. Bake 40-45 minutes, or until lightly browned, moist in the middle and when a fork or skewer comes out "clean".

Makes: 16 brownies
Preparation time: 15 minutes
Baking time: 45 minutes to 1 hr
Serving size: 1-2 brownies

Corn-Free* | ~~Nut and Seed-Free~~ | ~~Nut or Seed-Free~~ | **Soy-Free**

* Check labels

HINTS, TIPS AND SUBSTITUTIONS

If you choose to use the chocolate chips, you may find the chocolate sweetens the recipe just fine without the need for the maple sugar crystals.

If you prefer a brownie that is less moist, reduce the amounts of flax seed and water to 3 tablespoons and ⅜ cup, respectively.

Packaged carob chips may contain gluten and corn. To make your own carob chips, see page 184 for a stevia-sweetened option.

Cinnamon added to your taste combines well with these ingredients.

This recipe makes approximately 18 muffins. Muffins bake for about 15-20 minutes.

AMOUNT PER 1 BROWNIE SERVING: Calories 270; Calories from Fat 160; Total Fat 18g; Saturated Fat 2.5g; Trans Fat 0g; Cholesterol 0mg; Sodium 190mg; Total Carbohydrate 27g; Dietary Fiber 3g; Sugars 9g; Protein 4g; Vitamin C 4% DV; Calcium 6% DV; Iron 4% DV. *Recipe analyzed with almond flour, sunflower oil, maple sugar crystals and allergy-free chips containing organic cane sugar.*

This recipe also works well in a loaf pan, muffin pan or an 8-inch round cake pan.

THUMBPRINT COOKIES
(A.K.A. BUN IN OVEN COOKIES)

These cookies were inspired by Cynthia Lair and recipes for other jelly-filled cookies. The dough works well for "traditional" holiday cookies made into a variety of shapes using cookie cutters. Cookies may be topped with natural decorating colors (see the Appendix and Resources section on page 302), raisins, or vegan carob chips to make faces and designs to share with your loved ones.

2 cups gluten-free all-purpose baking mix

1½ cups almond meal flour (or 1 cup of almonds ground up from scratch)

2 tsp baking powder

¼ tsp sea or Himalayan salt

⅓ cup maple or coconut sugar crystals or xylitol (ground in coffee grinder) (*Yacon syrup or brown rice syrup can also be used, mixed with liquid ingredients.*)

3 Tbsp ground flax seed (ground in coffee grinder) plus ⅜ cup warm filtered water

⅓ cup organic unrefined walnut or sunflower oil or organic Earth Balance® spread

⅓ cup freshly-squeezed apple juice (or organic, unsweetened 100% juice)

2 tsp alcohol-free almond flavoring

1 tsp alcohol-free vanilla flavoring

1 tsp alcohol-free orange or lemon flavoring

Fruit spread of choice (preferably organic, without sweetener) or squares of organic high-cacao content chocolate or a dollop of one of the chocolate toppings (on pages 163-166) in the middle.

1. Preheat oven to 350°F. Lightly grease two cookie sheets with unrefined, virgin coconut oil.

2. Combine flour, almonds or almond flour, baking powder, salt and sweetener in a mixing bowl. Set aside.

3. In a separate bowl, mix flax/water mixture and set aside. In another bowl, combine the oil, juice, and extracts (and liquid syrup if using this instead of xylitol or maple sugar crystals). Once the wet ingredients are combined, add the flax/water mixture.

4. Add wet ingredients to dry and mix well, kneading a little. Dough will be firm, but moist and malleable.

5. With your hands or cookie cutters, shape tablespoon-sized amounts of dough into balls, hearts or shapes of your choice. *This dough rises a little but does not spread outward, so more cookies can fit on each cookie sheet.* (Dough can be stored in an airtight container in the refrigerator for a week and can also be frozen and thawed once before using.)

6. Once the dough is in the shape you wish, flatten each one slightly and indent cookie with your thumb (or a child's thumb) and put about ½ tsp fruit spread in the imprint. (If using a chocolate square, bake cookies first, then top with chocolate while cookies are warm. The *Decadent Chocolate Mousse* on page 243 and the chocolate toppings on pages 163-166 work well as a dollop in the center of each cookie. Chill cookies after adding toppings.)

7. Bake until edges are golden, about 15 minutes.

Makes: 24 cookies (Tbsp size) 40 cookies (½ Tbsp heart-shaped)

Preparation time: 20 minutes

Baking time: 15 minutes

Serving size: 2 cookies

Corn-Free* | ~~Nut and Seed-Free~~ | ~~Nut or Seed-Free~~ | **Soy-Free**

* Check labels

Hints, Tips and Substitutions

If you are sensitive to nuts, use a different flavoring and/or see the Coconut Bun in the Oven Cookies on page 180.

If you use a gluten-free flour mix, check to see if your mix contains baking powder. If it does, omit adding extra baking powder to the recipe.

If you are sensitive to soy, use the soy-free (red container) version of Earth Balance[R].

If you prefer a drier dough, add 6-8 tablespoons of warm water (instead of ⅜ cup) to the flax mixture to create your desired consistency.

AMOUNT PER 2 COOKIE SERVING: Calories 250; Calories from Fat 130; Total Fat 14g; Saturated Fat 1g; Trans Fat 0g; Cholesterol 0mg; Sodium 370mg; Total Carbohydrate 28g; Dietary Fiber 3g; Sugars 5g; Protein 6g; Calcium 6% DV; Iron 4% DV. *Recipe analyzed for tablespoon-sized cookies made from maple sugar crystals, blueberry fruit spread and sunflower oil.*

COCONUT BUN IN OVEN COOKIES

I created these cookies as a way for people to enjoy the Thumbprint cookies (see page 178) even if they are sensitive to nuts and seeds. Although these cookies call for coconut, they have a delightful flavor unlike macaroons.

2 cups gluten-free all-purpose baking mix

1 cup brown rice flour

1 cup unsweetened, unsulphured, shredded organic coconut

¼ cup xylitol (ground in coffee grinder) (*Can use maple or coconut sugar crystals if preferred.*)

½ tsp xanthan gum (or use guar gum if corn-sensitive)

4 Tbsp ground flax seed (ground in coffee grinder) plus ½ cup warm filtered water

⅓ cup + 1/16 cup organic unrefined walnut or sunflower oil

⅛ cup + ⅓ cup fresh apple juice (or unsweetened organic 100% juice)

2 tsp alcohol-free almond or other flavoring

1 tsp alcohol-free vanilla flavoring

1 tsp alcohol-free orange or lemon flavoring

½ tsp - 1 tsp alcohol-free coconut flavoring (to your taste)

¾ Tbsp agar flakes plus ⅜ cup of filtered water

1 tsp aluminum-free baking powder

Fruit spread of choice (preferably organic, without sweetener) or squares of organic high-cacao content chocolate or a dollop of one of the chocolate toppings (on pages 163-166) in the middle.

1. Preheat oven to 350°F. Lightly grease two cookie sheets with unrefined, virgin coconut oil.

2. Combine flour, coconut, sweetener and xanthan gum into a mixing bowl. Set aside.

3. In a small bowl, combine the flax with water and set aside. In another bowl, combine the oil, juice, and flavorings and then add the flax/water mixture.

4. Add wet ingredients to dry mixture. Mix well to form a dough-like consistency, kneading a little. Dough will be firm, but moist and malleable.

5. In a small saucepan, combine the agar flakes with ⅜ cup filtered water. Over low-medium heat, allow the agar flakes to dissolve, stirring occasionally. It should take about 8-12 minutes for the mixture to reach a pourable, syrupy consistency.

6. Add 1 tsp baking powder to the agar flake/water mixture. Stir. This mixture will foam and expand, so make sure your kids are watching! ☺ After about one minute, use a spoon to add the warm, foamy mixture to the dough (in step 4). Combine well.

7. With your hands or cookie cutters, shape tablespoon-sized amounts of dough into balls, hearts, moons or shapes of your choice. Drop cookies onto a lightly oiled cookie sheet. (*Dough can be stored in an airtight container in the refrigerator for a week and can also be frozen and thawed once before using.*)

8. Once the dough is in the shape you wish, flatten each one slightly and indent cookie with your thumb (or a child's thumb) and put about ½ tsp fruit spread in the imprint. (If using a chocolate square, bake cookies first, then top with chocolate while cookies are warm. The *Decadent Chocolate Mousse* on page 243 and the chocolate toppings on pages 163-166 work well as a dollop in the center of each cookie. Chill cookies after adding toppings.)

9. Bake until edges are golden, about 15 minutes.

Makes: 28 cookies
Preparation time: 30 minutes
Baking time: 15 minutes
Serving size: 2 cookies

Corn-Free* | ~~Nut and Seed-Free~~ | **Nut or Seed-Free** | **Soy-Free**

* Check labels

HINTS, TIPS AND SUBSTITUTIONS

If you are sensitive to nuts, choose a different flavoring to replace the almond.

AMOUNT PER 2 COOKIE SERVING: Calories 230; Calories from Fat 100; Total Fat 11g; Saturated Fat 3.5g Trans Fat 0g; Cholesterol 0mg; Sodium 230mg; Total Carbohydrate 31g; Dietary Fiber 2g; Sugars 3g;Protein 4g; Iron 2% DV. *Recipe analyzed with xylitol, sunflower oil and blueberry fruit spread.*

CHOCOLATE CHIP COOKIES

People have asked me for a version of the "real kind" of chocolate chip cookies. After many trials, I created these cookies, which are tasty like the more traditional "Toll House", but with significantly less sweetener. They are a good 'ole "stand-by" for holidays and parties.

3 Tbsp ground flax seed (ground in coffee grinder) plus ⅜ cup warm filtered water

1 tsp ground chia seeds (ground in coffee grinder) plus ⅛ cup warm filtered water

½ cup organic unrefined walnut or sunflower oil

2 tsp alcohol-free vanilla flavoring

¾ cup maple or coconut sugar crystals (ground in coffee grinder)

1 cup brown rice flour

1 cup millet flour

¼ cup gluten-free oat flour

½ Tbsp arrowroot flour

½ tsp baking soda

¼ tsp sea or Himalayan salt

¾ Tbsp agar flakes plus ⅜ cup of filtered water

1 tsp aluminum-free baking powder

¾ –1 cup fruit-sweetened, allergen- and dairy-free chocolate chips or vegan carob chips (*These chips may contain cane sugar.*)

1. Preheat oven to 350°F. Lightly grease two cookie sheets with unrefined, virgin coconut oil.

2. Combine the flax-water mixture and set aside. Combine the chia-water mixture and set aside.

3. In a large bowl, combine the oil and vanilla. Add the flax/water mixture and the chia/water mixture to these wet ingredients.

4. In a separate bowl, combine ground maple sugar crystals, flours, arrowroot, baking soda, and salt. Set aside.

5. Slowly add the dry flour mixture to the wet mixture until fully folded in, creating a dough-like consistency.

6. In a small saucepan, combine the agar flakes with ⅜ cup filtered water. Over low-medium heat, allow the agar flakes to dissolve, stirring occasionally. It should take about 8-12 minutes for the mixture to reach a pourable, syrupy consistency.

7. Add 1 tsp baking powder to the agar flake/water mixture. Stir. This mixture will foam and expand, so make sure your kids are watching! ☺ After about one minute, use a spoon to add the warm, foamy mixture to the dough (in step 5). Combine well. Fold in the chocolate chips.

8. Using a tablespoon, drop cookies onto a lightly oiled cookie sheet. (*This dough rises a little but does not spread outward, so more cookies can fit on each cookie sheet.*)

9. Bake for approximately 10-13 minutes, until soft and golden or slightly browned. Let the cookies cool on the cookie sheets before removing with a spatula. If you like a firmer cookie (as opposed to chewy and gooey), bake for several more minutes.

Makes: 30 cookies
Preparation time: 30 minutes
Baking time: 15-20 minutes
Serving Size: 2 cookies

Corn-Free* | ~~*Nut and Seed-Free*~~ | **Nut or Seed-Free** | **Soy-Free**

* Check labels

HINTS, TIPS AND SUBSTITUTIONS

Packaged carob chips may contain gluten and corn. To make your own carob chips, see page 184 for a stevia-sweetened option.

AMOUNT PER 2 COOKIE SERVING: Calories 210; Calories from Fat 110; Total Fat 13g; Saturated Fat 3g; Trans Fat 0g; Cholesterol 0mg; Sodium 100mg; Total Carbohydrate 23g; Dietary Fiber 2g; Sugars 9g; Protein 3g; Calcium 2% DV; Iron 4% DV. *Recipe analyzed with sunflower oil and 1 cup allergy-free chips containing organic cane sugar.*

CAROB CHIPS AND CAROB BARK

This recipe was inspired by Sally Fallon and Mary G. Enig's <u>Nourishing Traditions</u> recipe for carob chips.

The recipe may be made into chips, as a replacement for any of the chocolate chips noted in this book, or into carob bark, a stand-alone delicacy cut into flat, organic shapes. I have included this recipe since many vegan chocolate chips contain cane sugar, and store-bought carob chips may contain corn and gluten.

¾ cup carob powder

⅛ tsp stevia liquid or powder

1 cup unrefined, virgin coconut oil

1 Tbsp alcohol-free vanilla flavoring

1 tsp alcohol-free chocolate flavoring or chocolate stevia (optional)

1. Lightly oil a piece of parchment paper and place it into an 8 x 8 pan or loaf pan.

2. Combine ingredients in a bowl. Pour 1 cup of water into the saucepan and place the bowl of ingredients inside, creating a double boiler.

3. Heat ingredients until melted. Mix well with a spoon. Taste the mixture. If you prefer a sweeter flavor, add an extra ⅛ tsp stevia. *Using too much stevia will make the mixture taste bitter.*

4. Spread carob mixture onto the parchment paper. Refrigerate until cooled and hardened. Peel away paper. Cut into small chips or larger bark pieces. When coconut oil dries unevenly, the striations created between the hardened coconut oil and carob make the bark beautiful.

5. Store chips in the refrigerator in an airtight container.

Makes: 1 cup
Preparation time: 10 minutes
Waiting time: about 3-4 hours
Serving size: ⅛ cup or 2 Tbsp

Corn-Free | *Nut and Seed-Free* | *Nut or Seed-Free* | *Soy-Free*

HINTS, TIPS AND SUBSTITUTIONS

If you plan to prepare this recipe using chocolate flavoring, you may want to first check with the manufacturer of the chocolate flavoring to determine if the product is vegan.

AMOUNT PER ⅛ CUP OR 2 TBSP SERVING: Calories 300; Calories from Fat 240; Total Fat 28g; Saturated Fat 24g Trans Fat 0g; Cholesterol 0mg; Sodium 10mg; Total Carbohydrate 25g; Dietary Fiber 4g; Sugars 16g; Protein 2g; Iron 4% DV; Calcium 15% DV. *Recipe analyzed with stevia.*

For a picture of Carob Bark, see
www.SweetnessWithoutSugar.com.

BERRY BROWNIES

These are delicious and have everything! They have the smooth and gooey along with the occasional chip chunk. They are great as brownies or even mini cupcakes. You would never know that they contain so much fruit and so little additional sugar. My husband calls these "Awesome!"

1 cup pitted dates, ground into small pieces

1 cup prunes, ground into small pieces (Try with figs!)

1 cup frozen pitted cherries, ground into small pieces (*Drain extra water when thawed.*)

2 Tbsp ground flax seed (ground in coffee grinder) plus ¼ cup warm filtered water

1 cup gluten-free all purpose baking mix

1 cup brown rice flour

½ tsp xanthan gum (or use guar gum if corn-sensitive)

⅓ cup unsweetened, dairy-free cocoa powder or carob

⅔ cup pure maple syrup or less (unprocessed without added corn syrup or sweetener)

¼ cup organic unrefined walnut or sunflower oil or coconut oil

1 tsp alcohol-free vanilla flavoring

¼ cup fruit-sweetened, allergen- and dairy-free chocolate chips or vegan carob chips (*These chips may contain cane sugar.*)

1. Preheat oven to 350°F. Lightly grease an 8 x 8 pan with unrefined, virgin coconut oil.

2. With a Cuisinart[R] or high-speed blender, grind dates, prunes and cherries into small pieces. Transfer fruit into a separate bowl and combine with the rest of the ingredients.

3. Press/pour into an 8 x 8 pan, or spoon into muffin cups.

4. Bake for 20 minutes and check for doneness. If not quite done, reduce the oven temperature to 200°F and bake for another 10-15 minutes. Baking these for less time makes delicious, moist and hearty brownies.

5. Allow brownies to cool before cutting.

Makes: 16 brownies/28 mini muffins
Preparation time: 20 minutes
Baking time: 20-35 minutes
Serving size: 1-2 brownies or mini muffins

Corn-Free* | Nut and Seed-Free | Nut or Seed-Free | Soy-Free

* Check labels

HINTS, TIPS AND SUBSTITUTIONS

See the Appendix and Resources *section on page 306 for carob and dairy-free cocoa suggestions.*

Packaged carob chips may contain gluten and corn. To make your own carob chips, see page 184 for a stevia-sweetened option.

AMOUNT PER 1 BROWNIE SERVING: Calories 210; Calories from Fat 50; Total Fat 6g; Saturated Fat 1g; Trans Fat 0g; Cholesterol 0mg; Sodium 85mg; Total Carbohydrate 40g; Dietary Fiber 3g; Sugars 21g; Protein 3g; Vitamin A 4% DV; Vitamin C 2% DV; Iron 4% DV. *Recipe analyzed with walnut oil and allergy-free chips containing organic cane sugar.*

These also make nice mini muffins
or cupcakes.

DATE BARS

My friend, Jodie, brought these treats to my daughter's baby blessing celebration. They were sweet and satisfying, made with butter and yummy ingredients. With Jodie's permission I have made them gluten- and dairy-free and used alternative sweeteners.

FILLING:

2½ cups pitted dates (*May substitute sulfite-free figs or apricots.*)

½ cup filtered water (*Add more water as needed to reach a thickened consistency.*)

1. In a saucepan, simmer dates and water on low for about 10-15 minutes, stirring frequently, until the mixture thickens.

2. Cool the mixture by placing it in the refrigerator for about 15 minutes.

3. Using a food processor or hand mixer, blend date/water mixture into a spreadable consistency.

CRUST BOTTOM: (*For more details about this crust, please see page 216.*)

1½ cups gluten-free baking mix

1¾ cups gluten-free rolled oats

¼ cup maple or coconut sugar crystals (ground in coffee grinder)

1 cup organic, GMO-free Earth Balance® spread (2 sticks)

¾ Tbsp agar flakes plus ⅜ cup of filtered water

1 tsp aluminum-free baking powder

1. Preheat oven to 375°F. Lightly grease an 8 x 8 pan with unrefined, virgin coconut oil.

2. Mix together flour, oats and sweetener.

3. Melt the Earth Balance® and add it to the flour/oat mixture.

4. In a small saucepan, combine the agar flakes with ⅜ cup filtered water filtered water. Over low-medium heat, allow the agar flakes to dissolve, stirring occasionally. It should take about 8-12 minutes for the mixture to reach a pourable, syrupy consistency.

5. Add 1 tsp baking powder to the agar flake/water mixture. Stir. This mixture will foam and expand, so make sure your kids are watching!☺ After about one minute, use a spoon to add the warm, foamy mixture to the flour/oat mixture. Combine well.

6. Press half of the crust mixture into the bottom of the pan.

7. Spread the date mixture on top, pressing down to cover the bottom crust.

8. Add the remaining dry ingredients (crust mixture) to the top.

9. Bake for 20 minutes, until lightly browned.

10. Cut into square bars and serve.

Makes: 16 bars
Preparation time: 30 minutes
Baking time: 20 minutes
Serving size: 1 bar

Corn-Free | Nut and Seed-Free | Nut or Seed-Free | Soy-Free*

* Check labels

AMOUNT PER 1 BAR SERVING: Calories 280; Calories from Fat 110; Total Fat 12g; Saturated Fat 3.5g; Trans Fat 0g; Cholesterol 0mg; Sodium 240mg; Total Carbohydrate 41g; Dietary Fiber 4g; Sugars 19g; Protein 4g; Vitamin A 10% DV; Calcium 2% DV; Iron 4% DV. *Recipe analyzed with dates and* Jodie's Date Bar Crust *on page 216.*

If you are sensitive to soy, use the soy-free (red container) version of Earth Balance®.

QUINOA CHOCOLATE CHIP COOKIES

*We refer to these in our home as the "hockey puck cookies".
Their fiber, flax and chocolate combine to make these
treats not only tasty, but hearty, heart healthy, and fun.
They have a consistency similar to shortbread.*

This recipe is pictured on the cover.

1½ cups quinoa flakes

1 cup brown rice flour or millet flour

¼ tsp sea or Himalayan salt

2 Tbsp ground flax seed (ground in coffee grinder) plus ¼ cup warm
    filtered water

⅓ cup organic unrefined walnut or sunflower or coconut oil

⅓ cup pure maple syrup (unprocessed without added corn syrup or
    sweetener) or yacon or brown rice syrup

1 tsp alcohol-free vanilla flavoring

¾ Tbsp agar flakes plus ⅜ cup of filtered water

1 tsp aluminum-free baking powder

⅓ cup fruit-sweetened, allergen- and dairy-free chocolate chips or ⅓ cup
    vegan carob chips (*These chips may contain cane sugar.*)

1. Preheat oven to 350°F. Lightly grease two cookie sheets with unrefined, virgin coconut oil.

2. In a bowl, combine quinoa flakes, flour and salt. Set aside.

3. In a measuring cup or small bowl, combine the flax seed and water and set aside. In another bowl, mix together sweetener, oil, and vanilla. Combine both mixtures.

4. Add wet ingredients to dry mixture. Mix well to form a dough-like consistency.

5. In a small saucepan, combine the agar flakes with ⅜ cup filtered water. Over low-medium heat, allow the agar flakes to dissolve, stirring occasionally. It should take about 8-12 minutes for the mixture to reach a pourable, syrupy consistency.

6. Add 1 tsp baking powder to the agar flake/water mixture. Stir. This mixture will foam and expand, so make sure your kids are watching! ☺ After about one minute, use a spoon to add the warm, foamy mixture to the dough (in step 4). Combine well. Fold in the chocolate chips.

7. Using a teaspoon, drop cookies onto a lightly oiled cookie sheet.

8. Bake 15 minutes or until lightly browned.

Makes: 24 cookies
Preparation time: 25 minutes
Baking time: 15-20 minutes
Serving size: 1-2 cookies

Corn-Free* | Nut and Seed-Free | Nut or Seed-Free | Soy-Free

* Check labels

HINTS, TIPS AND SUBSTITUTIONS

People transitioning from refined sugar may wish to add a little more sweetener to suit their taste.

Packaged carob chips may contain gluten and corn. To make your own carob chips, see page 184 for a stevia-sweetened option.

If desired, these cookies can be made in a larger size.

AMOUNT PER 2 COOKIE SERVING (OR 1 LARGER, 3-INCH ROUND COOKIE):
Calories 190; Calories from Fat 80; Total Fat 9g; Saturated Fat 2g; Trans Fat 0g; Cholesterol 0mg; Sodium 75mg; Total Carbohydrate 25g; Dietary Fiber 2g; Sugars 9g; Protein 3g; Iron 2% DV. *Recipe analyzed with brown rice flour, pure maple syrup, walnut oil and sweetened vegan chocolate chips.*

COCONUT MACAROONS

Over the years, while teaching my "Sweetness" classes, I've received many requests for a macaroon recipe. Pat Leavitt, a personal chef living in the Charlottesville area, brought some macaroons to our home that were gooey and yummy. They were a challenge to recreate in a gluten-free, vegan form. Here is an option that is very tasty that I hope you and your loved ones will enjoy.

MACAROONS:

½ cup gluten-free flour (e.g. brown rice, millet or amaranth)

1 cup ground almonds (ground in a coffee grinder or in a blender with a dry blade attachment) or store-bought almond flour/meal

2 cups unsweetened, unsulphured shredded organic coconut

¼ cup unrefined, virgin coconut oil or organic, GMO-free, Earth Balance® spread, melted or to a spreadable consistency

1 tsp alcohol-free vanilla flavoring

¾ cup or less pure maple syrup (unprocessed without added corn syrup or sweetener) or yacon syrup or brown rice syrup (to taste)

¼ cup unsweetened organic canned coconut milk or unsweetened, dairy-free milk (e.g. almond, brown rice or hemp milk)

CHOCOLATE TOPPING:

Choose from toppings on pages 163-166. (My personal preference for this recipe is Wendy's Wonderful Chocolate Topping Sauce on page 163.)

1. Preheat oven to 350°F.

2. Mix the flour, ground almonds or almond meal, and coconut.

3. In a separate bowl, combine the oil or Earth Balance[R], vanilla, sweetener and coconut milk (or dairy-free milk).

4. Combine dry and wet mixtures. The final mixture should have a moist, sticky consistency. Press the mixture into an ungreased 8 x 8 pan.

5. Bake the macaroons for 15-20 minutes until lightly browned while preparing the chocolate sauce.

6. After cooling the macaroons until slightly warm to touch, top them with the chocolate sauce.

7. Chill macaroons for an hour or more before cutting into squares.

8. Because these macaroons tend to "go fast", you may wish to double the recipe, using a 13 x 9 x 2 baking pan.

Makes: 16 macaroons
Preparation time: 15 minutes
Baking time: 15-20 minutes
Serving size: 1 macaroon

Corn-Free | ~~Nut and Seed-Free~~ | ~~Nut or Seed-Free~~ | **Soy-Free**

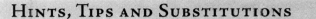

HINTS, TIPS AND SUBSTITUTIONS

If you are sensitive to soy, use the coconut oil or the soy-free (red container) version of Earth Balance®.

If you use less than ¾ cup sweetener, you may want to add more dairy-free milk to give macaroons a moist consistency.

AMOUNT PER 1 BAR SERVING: Calories 330; Calories from Fat 130; Total Fat 15g; Saturated Fat 10g; Trans Fat 0g; Cholesterol 0mg; Sodium 0mg; Total Carbohydrate 14g; Dietary Fiber 7g; Sugars 3g; Protein 3g; Vitamin C 20%DV; Calcium 2% DV; Iron 4% DV. *Recipe analyzed without chocolate topping and with millet flour, coconut oil, yacon syrup and full-fat unsweetened coconut milk.*

AMOUNT PER 1 BAR SERVING WITH *Wendy's Wonderful Chocolate Sauce:* Calories 410; Calories from Fat 190; Total Fat 22g; Saturated Fat 15g; Trans Fat 0g; Cholesterol 0mg; Sodium 0mg; Total Carbohydrate 21g; Dietary Fiber 8g; Sugars 9g; Protein 4g; Vitamin C 20%DV; Calcium 2% DV; Iron 6% DV. *Recipe analyzed with* Wendy's Wonderful Chocolate Sauce *from page 163.*

SPICY OATMEAL COOKIES

These cookies are an alternative to the traditional oatmeal cookie. With their warming spices, these bite-sized treats are a perfect snack with a hot cup of tea.

1 cup almond flour

1 cup hazelnut flour

1 cup gluten-free rolled oats

1 tsp ground cinnamon

½ tsp ground ginger powder

1 tsp ground cardamom

¼ tsp sea or Himalayan salt

1 Tbsp ground flax seed (ground in coffee grinder) plus ⅛ cup warm
   filtered water

½ cup walnut or sunflower oil

½ cup brown rice syrup or yacon syrup or liquid stevia to taste

½ tsp alcohol-free vanilla flavoring

½ tsp alcohol-free flavoring of choice (optional)

¾ Tbsp agar flakes plus ⅜ cup of filtered water

1 tsp aluminum-free baking powder

½ - ¾ cup raisins (optional)

1. Preheat oven to 350°F. Lightly grease cookie sheet with unrefined, virgin coconut oil.

2. In a large bowl, combine flours, oats, cinnamon, ginger, cardamom and salt.

3. Combine the flax seed with water and set aside. In a separate bowl, add the oil, sweetener, and flavorings. Add the flax/water mixture to the oil mixture. Stir until well combined.

4. Add the wet ingredients to the dry mixture. Mix well.

5. In a small saucepan, combine the agar flakes with ⅜ cup filtered water. Over low-medium heat, allow the agar flakes to dissolve, stirring occasionally. It should take about 8-12 minutes for the mixture to reach a pourable, syrupy consistency.

6. Add 1 tsp baking powder to the agar flake/water mixture. Stir to combine. This mixture will foam and expand, so make sure your kids are watching! ☺ After about one minute, use a spoon to add the warm, foamy mixture to the dough (in step 4).

7. Add raisins (if desired) and combine well.

8. Using a tablespoon, drop cookies onto a lightly oiled cookie sheet.

9. On a cookie sheet, place cookies one inch apart. Bake about 12 minutes or until bottoms are lightly browned.

10. Let cookies cool before removing them from baking sheet.

Makes: Approx. 24 cookies
Preparation time: 25 minutes
Baking time: 12-18 minutes
Serving size: 2 cookies

Corn-Free | ~~Nut and Seed-Free~~ | ~~Nut or Seed-Free~~ | **Soy-Free**

AMOUNT PER 2 COOKIE SERVING: Calories 300; Calories from Fat 180; Total Fat 21g; Saturated Fat 2g; Trans Fat 0g; Cholesterol 0mg; Sodium 95mg; Total Carbohydrate 26g; Dietary Fiber 3g; Sugars 11g; Protein 5g; Calcium 6% DV; Iron 8% DV. *Recipe analyzed with walnut oil, brown rice syrup and raisins.*

ALMOND CHOCOLATE CHIP COOKIES

We have also served these cookies as bon bons and they are usually gone in no time! Nut flour and citrus extract give this variation on the "traditional" chocolate chip cookie a lovely new texture and flavor. Many have asked for this recipe. I hope you like it too. A whole lot O' yum!

2 cups blanched almond flour or hazelnut flour

½ cup brown rice flour

1 tsp aluminum-free baking powder

½ tsp baking soda

¼ tsp sea or Himalayan salt

1 Tbsp ground flax seed (ground in coffee grinder) plus ⅛ cup warm
    filtered water

½ cup melted unrefined, virgin coconut oil (*Measured once melted.*)

½ cup brown rice syrup or yacon syrup

1 tsp alcohol-free vanilla flavoring

1 tsp alcohol-free orange or lemon or other flavoring

1 cup (or less) fruit-sweetened, allergen- and dairy-free chocolate chips or
    vegan carob chips (*These chips may contain cane sugar.*)

1. Preheat oven to 350°F. Lightly grease two cookie sheets with unrefined, virgin coconut oil.

2. In a large bowl, combine flours, baking powder, baking soda, and salt and set aside.

3. In a small measuring cup, combine the flax with water and set aside. Melt the coconut oil over low-medium heat in a small saucepan. In a small bowl whisk together the melted coconut oil, sweetener, and flavorings. Add the flax/water mixture to these wet ingredients.

4. Pour wet mixture into the dry mixture. With a spoon, mix the dough until well-combined. Dough will have a moist and sticky consistency.

5. Fold in the chocolate or carob chips.

6. Using a tablespoon, drop cookies onto a lightly-oiled cookie sheet. Leave space between the cookies to allow them to spread out during baking.

7. Bake 8-10 minutes or until bottoms are golden brown and tops are lightly brown. Allow them to cool completely before removing them from the baking sheet (preferably with a metal/stainless spatula). If you prefer to make them into bon bons, roll the baked cookies into a round bon bon and serve. *I have also made these cookies and added the agar flake and baking soda mixture (see steps 4 and 5 on page 189). Try making the cookies both ways to determine your preference.*

Makes: Approx. 24 cookies or bon bons
Preparation time: 25 minutes
Baking time: 8-10 minutes
Serving size: 2 cookies or bon bons

Corn-Free* | ~~*Nut and Seed-Free*~~ | ~~*Nut or Seed-Free*~~ | *Soy-Free*

* Check labels

HINTS, TIPS AND SUBSTITUTIONS

Packaged carob chips may contain gluten and corn. To make your own carob chips, see page 184 for a stevia-sweetened option. Omitting the chips in this recipe creates a light, citrus-flavored cookie.

These cookies work very well for making "ice cream sandwich" cookies with two cookies "sandwiching" ice cream in the middle.

Experiment without the chocolate chips and enjoy a "tea" cookie with a hint of citrus or other flavor of choice. These cookies or bon bons freeze well.

AMOUNT PER 2 COOKIE OR BON BON SERVING: Calories 340; Calories from Fat 210; Total Fat 24g; Saturated Fat 12g; Trans Fat 0g; Cholesterol 0mg; Sodium 200mg; Total Carbohydrate 31g; Dietary Fiber 3g; Sugars 15g; Protein 6g; Calcium 6% DV; Iron 4% DV. *Recipe analyzed with almond flour, brown rice syrup and allergy-free chips containing organic cane sugar.*

.

Frozen
Treats

Many of these recipes are pictured on my
website: *www.SweetnessWithoutSugar.com*

EASY FROZEN FRUIT TREAT

You may use fresh-squeezed juices from your favorite fruits (apple, mango, pear, pineapple, orange, etc.). This is a good recipe for people who are transitioning away from refined sugar and also craving a sweet treat. They are easy to make, easy to grab from the freezer and are free of dyes, unhealthy sweeteners and chemicals. The added oil helps to balance your blood sugar. These frozen treats also bring relief to teething babies.

FOR 8 (½ cup size) FROZEN TREATS (2 servings of fruit per treat):

> 4 cups unsweetened juice (e.g. preferably organic such as Lakewood[R] brand or fresh-squeezed juice)
>
> 2 tsp flax seed oil or hemp oil
>
> Add liquid stevia to taste before freezing. (*Do not use powdered stevia for this recipe.*)

FOR 1 (½ cup size) FROZEN TREAT (2 servings of fruit for a toddler):

> ½ cup unsweetened juice (e.g. preferably organic such as Lakewood[R] brand or fresh-squeezed juice)
>
> ¼ tsp flax seed oil or hemp oil
>
> Add liquid stevia to taste before freezing. (*Do not use powdered stevia for this recipe.*)

FOR 1 (¼ cup size) FROZEN TREAT (1 serving of fruit for a toddler):

> ¼ cup unsweetened juice (e.g. preferably organic such as Lakewood[R] brand or fresh-squeezed juice)
>
> ¼ cup filtered water
>
> ¼ tsp flax seed oil or hemp oil
>
> Add liquid stevia to taste before freezing. (*Do not use powdered stevia for this recipe.*)

1. Using a blender, combine ingredients to help emulsify the oil.

2. Add liquid stevia to taste. Re-blend.

3. Pour contents into ice pop molds and freeze for four hours or more.

Makes: 8 standard-size frozen treats (using ice pop molds)
Preparation time: 10 minutes or less
Freezing time: 4 hours or more
Serving size: 1 frozen treat

Corn-Free | Nut and Seed-Free | **Nut or Seed-Free** | **Soy-Free**

Hints, Tips and Substitutions

The "standard size" single treat holds a half cup of liquid. These are the size of a push-pop or half the size of a "wide" Fudgicle®. These molds are often sold in sets of four. This recipe will prepare enough frozen treats for two sets.

If sensitive to nuts and seeds, substitute with a different oil.

If trying these treats with your teething baby, I suggest using a fruit your child has handled well and enjoyed.

This recipe can be enjoyed if you are following a raw diet. For more raw recipes, please see pages 247-291.

AMOUNT PER 1 (½ CUP) FROZEN TREAT SERVING (OF 2 FRUIT PER SERVING VERSION): Calories 60; Calories from Fat 10; Total Fat 1g; Saturated Fat 0g; Trans Fat 0g; Cholesterol 0mg; Sodium 0mg; Total Carbohydrate 13g; Dietary Fiber 1g; Sugars 12g; Protein 1g. *Recipe analyzed with store-bought organic, unsweetened apple juice and flax oil.*

FRUITY FROZEN YOGURT

This yogurt contains sugar, so this is a refreshing, creamy, vegan treat to enjoy occasionally. This recipe is wonderful for vegans (and non-vegans) who seek delicious alternatives to ice cream, Popsicles® and frozen yogurt. This can also be eaten instantly, like a smoothie, or as a topping over cereal.

2 cups organic raspberries or blueberries

1½ Tbsp fresh lemon juice

Liquid stevia to taste

½ cup So Delicious® coconut plain yogurt or Ricera® yogurt

½ cup unsweetened, dairy-free milk (e.g. almond, brown rice or hemp milk)

¼ cup coconut *cream* (not oil)

1. Pureé raspberries and lemon juice. If desired, strain out the seeds using a fine mesh strainer.

2. Add liquid stevia to taste.

3. Blend raspberries and lemon with the rest of the ingredients.

4. Pour into a freezer-safe container or into ice pop molds. If you want a creamier texture, thaw the mixture until soft, but not thoroughly melted, then re-blend the mixture. Refreeze the second blending and serve when ready to eat.

Makes: 2 cups (about 4 standard-size ice pops)
Preparation time: 10 minutes or less
Freezing time: 4 hours or more
Serving size: ½ cup or 1 ice pop

Corn-Free* | Nut and Seed-Free | Nut or Seed-Free | Soy-Free

* Check labels

HINTS, TIPS AND SUBSTITUTIONS

Raspberries (especially frozen ones) can be tart. More stevia may be needed to suit your taste.

If you tolerate soy, you may also use Wildwood™ or Whole Soy & Co.® soy yogurts for a higher protein content. Coconut milk (unsweetened) makes a delicious substitute.

For a raw version of this recipe, please see page 276.

AMOUNT PER ½ CUP SERVING OR 1 ICE POP: Calories 110; Calories from Fat 70; Total Fat 7g; Saturated Fat 6g; Trans Fat 0g; Cholesterol 0mg; Sodium 5mg; Total Carbohydrate 13g; Dietary Fiber 1g; Sugars 2g; Protein 2g; Vitamin C 25%; Calcium 6% DV; Iron 6% DV. *Recipe analyzed with raspberries, So Delicious® plain coconut yogurt and unsweetened hemp milk.*

CREAMY ORANGE ICE POP

Enjoy this frozen confection reminiscent of the "oldie but goodie".
This version contains fiber, Vitamin C, protein, fat and sugar from
fresh oranges only! This can be part of a meal from a parents' point
of view and a treat from a kids' perspective. Everybody's happy.

2 seedless oranges, peeled and de-seeded

1 cup plain, unsweetened soy probiotic yogurt (e.g. Wildwood Organics™)

¼ cup plus ⅛ cup of orange juice, packaged or freshly-squeezed (juice
  from 1 medium orange)

5 Tbsp coconut *cream* (not oil)

5 tsp alcohol-free vanilla flavoring

12-15 drops SteviaClear ᴿ Vanilla Crème flavor (*Add more to suit your taste.*)

1. In a blender, blend together all ingredients (on high) until smooth. If desired,
   blend for less time to retain the "pulpy" texture.

2. Pour into the ice pop molds or ice cube trays. Freeze for 4 hours or more. *Fills
   approximately 1¼ ice cube trays.*

Makes: 6 thin ½ cup molded ice pops
Preparation time: 10 minutes or less
Freezing time: 4 hours or more
Serving size: 1 ice pop or 3 cubes

Corn-Free* | *Nut and Seed-Free* | *Nut or Seed-Free* | *Soy-Free*

* Check labels

HINTS, TIPS AND SUBSTITUTIONS

To replace the Wildwood Organics™ yogurt above, try any one of these four substitutions:

1 package of organic (vacuum packed) silken tofu (contains soy)
1 cup So Delicious® plain coconut yogurt (soy-free; contains cane sugar)
1 cup Ricera® rice-based yogurt (soy-free; contains cane sugar)
1 cup unsweetened coconut milk

Preferable to choose organic juice; Flavor will vary with different brands of packaged orange juices.

For a raw version of this recipe, please see page 278.

AMOUNT PER 1 (½ CUP) ICE POP SERVING: Calories 100; Calories from Fat 45; Total Fat 5g; Saturated Fat 4g; Trans Fat 0g; Cholesterol 0mg; Sodium 10mg; Total Carbohydrate 11g; Dietary Fiber 3g; Sugars 5g; Protein 2g; Vitamin A 2% DV; Vitamin C 50% DV; Calcium 8% DV; Iron 4% DV. *Recipe analyzed with Wildwood Organics™ plain yogurt.*

CHOCOLATE FUDGE ICE POP

This recipe tastes wonderful in cold or warm weather. I've worked with people who get excited about having a low-fat, artificially-sweetened or sugar-laden frozen treat for a night-time snack. This tasty ice pop alternative, containing protein and healthy fat (to offset the natural fruit sugar) will provide satiety and satisfy your sweet tooth!

½ cup plain, unsweetened soy probiotic yogurt (e.g. Wildwood Organics™)

4 Tbsp unsweetened, dairy-free cocoa powder or carob powder

⅔ cup unsweetened, dairy-free milk (e.g. almond, brown rice or hemp milk)

2 Tbsp coconut *cream* (not oil; optional) (*Adds to the smooth consistency.*)

1 tsp alcohol-free vanilla flavoring

1 banana

3 pitted dates, optional

Liquid stevia to suit your taste

1. Combine all ingredients in a blender. Blend well.

2. Add liquid stevia to your taste.

3. Pour into the ice pop mold or ice cube trays. Freeze for 4 hours or more. *Fills approximately 1¼ ice cube trays.* Enjoy!

Makes: 6 thin ½ cup molded ice pops
Preparation time: 10 minutes or less
Freezing time: 4 hours or more
Serving size: 1 ice pop or 3 cubes

Corn-Free* | Nut and Seed-Free | Nut or Seed-Free | Soy-Free

* Check labels

HINTS, TIPS AND SUBSTITUTIONS

To replace the Wildwood Organics™ yogurt above, try any one of these three substitutions:
½ cup organic silken tofu (boxed or refrigerated; contains soy)
½ cup So Delicious® coconut yogurt (soy-free; contains cane sugar)
½ cup Ricera® rice-based yogurt (soy-free; contains cane sugar)

See the Appendix and Resources section on pages 300-306 for dairy-free cocoa, milk and yogurt suggestions.

You may replace the dairy-free milk with unsweetened dairy-free chocolate milk.

Amount per 1 (½ cup) ice pop serving: Calories 80; Calories from Fat 35; Total Fat 3.5g; Saturated Fat 1.5g; Trans Fat 0g; Cholesterol 0mg; Sodium 10mg; Total Carbohydrate 9g; Dietary Fiber 3g; Sugars 4g; Protein 2g; Vitamin C 4%; Calcium 4% DV; Iron 6% DV. *Recipe analyzed with Wildwood Organics™ soy plain yogurt, unsweetened hemp milk, coconut cream and dates.*

"MILK" SHAKE

This is so easy to make! It tastes like a regular milkshake and contains protein! When flavoring with chocolate or vanilla protein powder, you can't go wrong. Great for kids of all ages.

1 cup unsweetened dairy-free milk (e.g. almond, brown rice or hemp milk)

2-3 bananas, frozen

2 cups filtered water

Chocolate- or vanilla-flavored protein powder (choose one):
   ¼ cup (1 scoop) Nutribiotic® Rice Protein, or
   ⅛ cup (1 scoop) Raw Power!™ Protein Superfood Supplement®, or
   ¼ cup (1 scoop) Sun Warrior Protein®

1. Combine ingredients in a blender until smooth. Add enough liquid to create your preferred consistency.

2. Pour into a glass, serve and enjoy.

Makes: 4 cups
Preparation time: 10 minutes
Serving size: 1 cup

Corn-Free | *Nut and Seed-Free* | *Nut or Seed-Free* | *Soy-Free*

HINTS, TIPS AND SUBSTITUTIONS

For more protein, add more powder to your glass or drink more than one cup. It's easy!

Raw Power!™ Protein Superfood Supplement® contains nuts. Substitute a different protein powder if making a nut-free version.

For a raw version of this recipe, please see page 279.

AMOUNT PER 1 CUP SERVING: Calories 160; Calories from Fat 20; Total Fat 2.5g; Saturated Fat 0g; Trans Fat 0g; Cholesterol 0mg; Sodium 20 mg; Total Carbohydrate 22g; Dietary Fiber 3g; Sugars 12g; Protein 14g; Vitamin A 2% DV; Vitamin C 15% DV; Calcium 2% DV; Iron 6% DV. *Recipe analyzed using unsweetened hemp milk, 3 bananas and Nutribiotic Brown Rice Protein®.*

Muffins,
Pies and Crisps

Many of these recipes are pictured on my
website: *www.SweetnessWithoutSugar.com*

QUINOA FRUIT MUFFINS

These muffins are dense and hearty. People who have been "off" sugar for a while will enjoy the sweetness the fruit provides. Our son, Solomon, likes these "cold", right out of the "friggerator." Can also be warmed and eaten with oil, Earth Balance® and/or stevia drops.

1 cup quinoa flakes

1 cup millet flour

4 tsp baking powder

2 tsp baking soda

¾ tsp xanthan gum (or use guar gum if corn-sensitive)

½ tsp sea or Himalayan salt

1 Tbsp unrefined, virgin coconut oil, melted

3 Tbsp ground flax seed (ground in coffee grinder) plus ⅜ cup warm
    filtered water

1 tsp ground chia seeds (ground in coffee grinder) plus ⅛ cup warm
    filtered water

4 Tbsp pure maple syrup (unprocessed without added corn syrup or
    sweetener)

2 ripe bananas, mashed

1 generous cup berries (*Frozen berries work well, but may require a longer
    baking time.*)

1. Preheat oven to 400°F. Lightly grease a 12-muffin pan.

2. Combine quinoa flakes, flour, baking powder, baking soda, xanthan gum and salt. Set aside.

3. Melt the coconut oil over low-medium heat in a small saucepan. In a small bowl, combine the flax-water mixture and set aside. In another small bowl, combine the chia-water mixture and set aside.

4. In a separate bowl, mix together melted coconut oil, flax seed mixture, chia seed mixture, sweetener, mashed bananas, and berries.

5. Add wet ingredients to dry mixture and mix well.

6. Spoon muffin mixture into muffin pan.

7. Bake for 20-25 minutes, until a toothpick inserted in the center comes out clean.

Makes: 12 large or 18 smaller muffins
Preparation time: 15 minutes
Baking time: 20-25 minutes for all sizes
Serving size: 1 muffin

Corn-Free | *Nut and Seed-Free* | *Nut or Seed-Free* | *Soy-Free*

Hints, Tips and Substitutions

Other non-gluten flours such as brown rice or quinoa work well in this recipe. If you use either of these flours, you may want to add 1-2 more tablespoons of sweetener to suit your taste.

For a similar final product with a drier texture, omit the xanthan gum and chia seed mixture and use only 3 tablespoons ground flax seed plus ⅜ cup warm filtered water.

For more muffin ideas, see the Cakes and Cupcakes section. Also, the "Bready" Banana Brownies (see page 176) and Berry Brownies (see page 186) recipes make excellent muffins.

AMOUNT PER 1 LARGE MUFFIN SERVING (ONE OF TWELVE): Calories 130; Calories from Fat 25; Total Fat 3g; Saturated Fat 1g; Trans Fat 0g; Cholesterol 0mg; Sodium 450mg; Total Carbohydrate 25g; Dietary Fiber 3g; Sugars 8g; Protein 3g; Vitamin C 4%; Calcium 4% DV; Iron 4% DV. *Recipe analyzed with millet flour, pure maple syrup and blueberries.*

WENDY'S NUT-FREE PIE CRUST

This crust works well for bars and for pies. It is tasty, easy and doesn't take long to make. It has a denser flavor than a traditional flaky pie crust. It can hold a variety of fillings without becoming soggy.

½ cup organic unrefined walnut or sunflower oil (*Coconut oil also works well.*)

¼ cup (or less to taste) brown rice syrup or yacon or pure maple syrup (unprocessed without added corn syrup or sweetener)

1 cup gluten-free baking mix

1½ cups quinoa flakes

¼ -½ tsp sea or Himalayan salt

1 tsp cinnamon

¾ Tbsp agar flakes plus ⅜ cup of filtered water

1 tsp aluminum-free baking powder

1. Preheat oven to 350°F. Lightly grease an 8- or 9-inch pie pan with unrefined oil.

2. Using a spoon, mix together oil and sweetener. Add the flour mix, quinoa flakes, salt, and cinnamon. Continue to mix with a spoon (or with your hands) until the mixture forms into a dough-like consistency.

3. In a small saucepan, combine the agar flakes with ⅜ cup filtered water. Over low-medium heat, allow the agar flakes to dissolve, stirring occasionally. This takes about 8-12 minutes to reach a pourable, syrupy consistency. Once the flakes are dissolved, add the teaspoon of baking powder and stir until combined and fully foamed. With a spoon, stir the foamy agar mixture into the crust ingredients. Mix until well-combined.

4. Press mixture into greased 8- or 9-inch round cake or pie pan. You may wish to save some mixture for a lattice topping. Pressing all the mixture into the bottom of the pan makes a thick crust (sometimes more crust than pie). For a deeper crust that lines the sides of the pan, make a little extra mixture. If you are making bars, press the crust into an 8 x8 pan instead.

5. Bake the crust for 10-15 minutes until set.

Makes: 1 crust for 8- or 9-inch round cake or pie pan
Preparation time: 25 minutes
Baking time: 10-15 minutes
Serving size: 1 slice

Corn-Free* | *Nut and Seed-Free* | *Nut or Seed-Free* | *Soy-Free*

* Check labels

HINTS, TIPS AND SUBSTITUTIONS

Different gluten-free flours can sometimes cause the sweetener and oil to pool together in this "dough". If after you press the mixture into the pan/plate, the dough has a "wet" consistency, use a paper towel to blot it and bake it to set. If there is additional pooling after baking, blot it again before adding the topping. This will not affect the final product.

AMOUNT PER 1 SLICE OF 8 SERVING: Calories 300; Calories from Fat 130; Total Fat 15g; Saturated Fat 1.5g; Trans Fat 0g; Cholesterol 0mg; Sodium 290mg; Total Carbohydrate 38g; Dietary Fiber 2g; Sugars 6g; Protein 4g; Calcium 2% DV. *Recipe analyzed with sunflower oil, brown rice syrup and ¼ tsp sea salt.*

WENDY'S PIE CRUST WITH NUTS

This crust also works well for bars and for pies. Like the nut-free pie crust on page 212, this crust is delicious and easy to make. It has a rich flavor with a dense consistency. It also holds a variety of fillings without becoming soggy.

1 cup quinoa flakes

½ cup raw hazelnuts, almonds or walnuts (or their flours)

½ cup gluten-free baking mix

⅓ cup organic unrefined walnut or sunflower oil

2 Tbsp brown rice syrup or pure maple syrup (unprocessed without
      added corn syrup or sweetener)

¾ Tbsp agar flakes plus plus ⅜ cup of filtered water

1 tsp aluminum-free baking powder

1. Preheat oven to 350°F. Lightly grease an 8- or 9-inch pie pan with unrefined oil.

2. Blend quinoa flakes and nuts in a food processor until finely chopped.

3. In a mixing bowl, combine quinoa flake/nut mixture with flour.

4. In a separate bowl, combine oil, sweetener and water.

5. Mix wet ingredients with dry. In a small saucepan, combine the agar flakes with ⅜ cup filtered water. Over low-medium heat, allow the agar flakes to dissolve, stirring occasionally. This takes about 8-12 minutes to reach a pourable, syrupy consistency. Once the flakes are dissolved, add the teaspoon of baking powder and stir until well-combined and foamy.

6. With a spoon, add the foamy agar mixture to the wet/dry mixture and combine well. *Mixture may be slightly wet and crumbly.*

7. You may press the mixture onto the bottom of the pan, or onto the bottom and sides. Bake crust for 10-12 minutes. Remove from oven and allow to cool.

Makes: 1 crust for 8- or 9-inch round cake or pie pan
Preparation time: 25 minutes
Baking time: 10-15 minutes
Serving size: 1 slice

Corn-Free* | ~~*Nut and Seed-Free*~~ | ~~*Nut or Seed-Free*~~ | *Soy-Free*

* Check labels

HINTS, TIPS AND SUBSTITUTIONS

Different gluten-free flours can sometimes cause the sweetener and oil to pool together in this "dough". If after you press the mixture into the pan/plate, the dough has a "wet" consistency, use a paper towel to blot it and bake it to set. If there is additional pooling after baking, blot it again before adding the topping. This will not affect the final product.

AMOUNT PER 1 SLICE OF 8 SERVING: Calories 240; Calories from Fat 130; Total Fat 15g; Saturated Fat 1.5g; Trans Fat 0g; Cholesterol 0mg; Sodium 160mg; Total Carbohydrate 23g; Dietary Fiber 2g; Sugars 4g; Protein 5g; Calcium 4% DV; Iron 2% DV. *Recipe analyzed with almonds, sunflower oil and brown rice syrup.*

JODIE'S DATE BAR CRUST

This crust is softer than those with and without nuts (as noted on pages 212-215). It has a crumbly consistency that holds its shape when pressed into the pan. Not only does this crust have a rich flavor, but it's also versatile and easy to make.

1½ cups gluten-free baking mix or flour

1¾ cups gluten-free rolled oats

¼ cup maple or coconut sugar crystals (ground in coffee grinder)

1 cup organic, GMO-free Earth Balance® spread (2 sticks)

¾ Tbsp agar flakes plus ⅜ cup filtered water

1 tsp aluminum-free baking powder

1. Preheat oven to 375°F. Grease an 8- or 9-inch cake or pie pan with unrefined, virgin coconut oil.

2. Mix together flour, oats and ground maple or coconut sugar crystals.

3. In a saucepan, melt the Earth Balance® spread. Stir into the flour/oat mixture.

4. Use a spoon or your hands to mix the ingredients into a dough-like consistency.

5. In a small saucepan, combine the agar flakes with ⅜ cup filtered water. Over low-medium heat, allow the agar flakes to dissolve, stirring occasionally. This takes about 8-12 minutes to reach a pourable, syrupy consistency. Once the flakes are dissolved, add the teaspoon of baking powder and stir until well-combined and foamy.

6. With a spoon, add the foamy agar mixture to the dough mixture and combine well.

7. Press the crust mixture into an 8- or 9-inch pie pan.

8. Bake for 10 minutes until it's set, then add filling and re-bake as noted in the recipe you are making.

Makes: 1 crust for 8- or 9-inch round cake or pie pan
Preparation time: 15 minutes
Baking time: 10 minutes
Serving size: 1 slice

Corn-Free* | *Nut and Seed-Free* | *Nut or Seed-Free* | *Soy-Free*

* Check labels

HINTS, TIPS AND SUBSTITUTIONS

*If you are sensitive to soy, use the soy-free (red container) version of Earth Balance*ᴿ*.*

AMOUNT PER 1 SLICE OF 16 SERVING: Calories 200; Calories from Fat 110; Total Fat 12g; Saturated Fat 3.5g; Trans Fat 0g; Cholesterol 0mg; Sodium 240mg; Total Carbohydrate 20g; Dietary Fiber 1g; Sugars 1g; Protein 3g; Vitamin A 10% DV; Calcium 2% DV; Iron 4% DV.

NUTTER NUMMY PIE

I've included this recipe twice because it's delicious in both pie and bar form. It's also easy to make with relatively few ingredients.

PIE CRUST BOTTOM:

Select a crust recipe on pages 212-217.

NUTTY FILLING:

1½ cups unsweetened and unsalted almond, cashew, hempseed or Brazil nut butter

½ cup ground xylitol (*Can substitute with ground maple or coconut sugar crystals.*)

¾ tsp sea or Himalayan salt

1½ cups unsweetened, dairy-free milk (e.g. almond, brown rice or hemp milk), plain variety

1 tsp alcohol-free vanilla flavoring (optional)

CHOCOLATE TOPPING:

Choose from toppings on pages 163-166.

1. Prepare crust as noted on pages 212-217. Pre-bake to set the crust.

2. In a saucepan over medium-high heat, combine nut butter, ground sweetener, salt, vanilla and dairy-free milk. Stir until mixed together. Do not boil. Pour mixture over baked crust. Allow to cool in the refrigerator for 1 hour.

3. While the pie cools, prepare a chocolate topping (if desired) noted on pages 163-166. Cover the pie with topping or drizzle a design over the top of the pie and set aside some topping that individuals can enjoy with their pie any way they like.

Makes: 16 slices; 1 (8-9 inch) pie
Preparation time: 25 minutes
Baking time: 15-20 minutes for crust; 25 minutes for filled pie
Chill and cool time: 1 hour or more
Serving size: 1 slice

Corn-Free* | ~~Nut and Seed-Free~~ | **Nut or Seed-Free** | **Soy-Free**

* Check labels

HINTS, TIPS AND SUBSTITUTIONS

To balance the sweet and salty flavors present in the topping and crust, you may prefer to add less salt to the filling.

Adding vanilla to this recipe will make the topping slightly brown. This will occur when using either vanilla flavoring or dairy-free unsweetened milk containing vanilla.

AMOUNT PER 1 SLICE OF 16 SERVING: Calories 310; Calories from Fat 190; Total Fat 22g; Saturated Fat 1.5g; Trans Fat 0g; Cholesterol 0mg; Sodium 150mg; Total Carbohydrate 24g; Dietary Fiber 4g; Sugars 3g; Protein 9g; Calcium 10% DV; Iron 10% DV. *Recipe analyzed using almond milk, xylitol and hemp milk for the filling and the Loco for Choco Sauce on page 166 and Wendy's Pie Crust with Nuts on page 214.*

Different nut butters and nut butter brands have different consistencies when heated or refrigerated. If your filling is "runnier" than desired, use a little more nut butter. Adding about 1 teaspoon or less of arrowroot starch will also help thicken the nut mixture upon heating.

COCONUT AND CREAMY PIE

This recipe was inspired by Ann Gentry's The Real Food Daily Cookbook recipe for coconut cream pie. It gets rave reviews whenever I bring it to a gathering. Traditional coconut cream pie is one of my brother-in-law's favorites, and he loves this new version. In our house, we've enjoyed this treat for dessert, a snack, and even breakfast.

PIE CRUST BOTTOM:

Select a crust recipe on pages 212-217.

CREAMY COCONUT FILLING:

1½ pounds extra-firm organic silken tofu (approximately 2 boxes)

½ cup maple or coconut sugar crystals and ½ cup xylitol (both ground in coffee grinder)

¾ cup unsweetened organic canned coconut milk

⅓ cup organic unrefined walnut or sunflower oil (*Coconut oil also works well.*)

3 Tbsp arrowroot

½ tsp alcohol-free almond flavoring (*Those sensitive to nuts may use coconut or other flavoring.*)

1¼ tsp alcohol-free vanilla flavoring

¼ tsp sea or Himalayan salt

¾ cup unsweetened, unsulphured shredded organic coconut

CHOCOLATE TOPPING:

Choose from toppings noted on pages 163-166.

1. Preheat oven to 350°F. Prepare crust as noted on pages 212-217. Pre-bake to set the crust.

2. In a blender or food processor, add the tofu, sweeteners, coconut milk, oil, arrowroot, almond and vanilla flavorings, sea salt and ½ cup of the shredded coconut. Blend or process until smooth and creamy. Then pour the blended mixture onto the baked pie crust.

3. Bake for 25 minutes. Remove from oven and evenly sprinkle the remaining ¼ cup shredded coconut over the pie. Bake the pie again until the coconut slightly browns and when the pan is gently shaken, the filling is

set (usually about 10-15 minutes). The center may still move even when the edges are set but will firm up once cooled. Allow the pie to cool before covering. Refrigerate for 4 hours, or until cold.

4. While the pie cools, prepare a chocolate topping (if desired) noted on pages 163-166.

5. Cut the pie into 16 slices and serve plain or, if desired, drizzled with chocolate sauce.

Makes: 16 slices; 1 (8-9 inch) pie
Preparation time: 15 minutes
Baking time: 15 - 20 minutes for crust 25 + 15 minutes for filled pie
Serving size: 1 slice

Corn-Free* | ~~Nut and Seed-Free~~ | *Nut or Seed-Free* | ~~Soy-Free~~

* Check labels

HINTS, TIPS AND SUBSTITUTIONS

We have used this recipe to make "eggs" for Easter. The coconut "cream" filling will fill approximately 20 plastic eggs. Prepare the filling only, bake for about 40 minutes, let it cool and then refrigerate it prior to filling the two sides of the plastic egg. Return the filled "egg" to the refrigerator until served. When kept refrigerated, batter will mold into the egg shape and delight kids of any age. If not sensitive to nuts, a baby-sized spoonful of nut butter can be added between the two "layers" of the egg to create a "yolk".

We use less sweetener in our version and often eat it without the sauce. It is still delicious!

AMOUNT PER 1 SLICE OF 16 SERVING: Calories 440; Calories from Fat 230; Total Fat 27g; Saturated Fat 6g; Trans Fat 0g; Cholesterol 0mg; Sodium 190mg; Total Carbohydrate 49g; Dietary Fiber 5g; Sugars 17g; Protein 8g; Calcium 8% DV; Iron 10% DV. *Recipe analyzed using ½ cup maple sugar crystals, ½ cup xylitol, full-fat coconut milk and Vanilla Chocolate Sauce on page 164 and Wendy's Pie Crust with Nuts on page 214.*

Though this recipe creates a decadent pie (or mini muffin pies), you can create equally delicious alternatives by omitting the chocolate sauce (or using less), using light coconut milk, and/or more xylitol instead of maple or coconut sugar crystals. Or, (though it's not as much fun), cut a smaller slice.

APPLE, PEAR OR BERRY CRISP

This recipe was adapted from one I experimented with during my days at Bastyr University. When made with pears and cashews this dessert is great for people who suspect they have food allergies. Very similar to the original Bastyr recipe, this version brings back one of many fond memories of our time in Seattle.

1 cup gluten-free flour (brown rice, amaranth, millet; can use ½ cup of
> two different flours)

½ tsp sea or Himalayan salt

¼ cup organic unrefined walnut or sunflower oil (*Coconut oil also works well.*)

Pure maple syrup (unprocessed without added corn syrup or sweetener)
> or yacon or brown rice syrup

⅓ cup macadamia nuts or cashews, blended or chopped well

2 Tbsp filtered water

2 Tbsp pure maple syrup (unprocessed without added corn syrup or
> sweetener) or yacon or brown rice syrup

2 tsp alcohol-free vanilla flavoring

5 cups peeled and sliced apple or pear (about 4-5 apples or pears, or 2-3
> cups of berries)

1. Preheat oven to 350ºF. Grease an 8 x 8 baking pan with unrefined, virgin coconut oil.

2. Mix flour and salt in a bowl. Add oil and ¼ cup sweetener and mix well. Using a coffee grinder, blend the nuts into small pieces or into a "powder" texture. Add ground nuts to the flour mixture and set aside.

3. In a small bowl, combine water, 2 tablespoons sweetener syrup and vanilla. Set aside.

4. Slice fruit and place into a lightly oiled 8 x 8 baking pan.

5. Pour the liquid mixture over the fruit and toss gently.

6. Spoon the flour-nut mixture over the top of the fruit. Spread the mixture evenly.

7. Cover and bake 45 minutes.

8. Uncover and bake 15 minutes more to brown the topping.

Makes: 8 servings
Preparation time: 20 minutes
Baking time: 45 minutes to 1 hour
Serving size: ½ - ¾ cup

Corn-Free | ~~Nut and Seed-Free~~ | **Nut or Seed-Free** | **Soy-Free**

HINTS, TIPS AND SUBSTITUTIONS

The sweetener in this recipe can also be replaced with stevia. Begin with 5 drops of stevia and add more to suit your taste.

If you are sensitive to nuts, use sunflower, hemp or pumpkin seeds. If sensitive to both nuts and seeds, use flour mixture only.

May wish to make more "flour-nut mixture" to add on top.

For breakfast, you may want to try a serving of fruit crisp with a tablespoon of brown rice protein powder. Warm it up and drizzle with a tablespoon of flax or hemp oil. For dessert, serve fruit crisp plain or enjoy it with dairy-free "ice cream", a dollop of coconut "ice cream", yogurt or Ricera® yogurt.

AMOUNT PER ½ CUP SERVING: Calories 230; Calories from Fat 100; Total Fat 12g; Saturated Fat 1.5g; Trans Fat 0g; Cholesterol 0mg; Sodium 85mg; Total Carbohydrate 32g; Dietary Fiber 3g; Sugars 18g; Protein 2g; Vitamin C 6% DV; Calcium 2% DV; Iron 4% DV. *Recipe analyzed with brown rice flour, walnut oil, macadamia nuts, pure maple syrup, apples, and without protein powder.*

RHUBARB BERRY CRISP

My mother-in-law once brought a traditional version of this recipe when she came to visit. I later made it vegan and gluten-free and we all enjoyed a delightful dinner and dessert together.

FILLING:

4 cups rhubarb, (about 5-6 long stalks) cut into small pieces

4 cups berries (*Strawberries are delicious in this recipe. If used, slice them in half. 4 cups = about 1 ½ lbs. or two 16-oz. containers.*)

¼ - ½ cup either brown rice syrup, pure maple syrup (unprocessed without added corn syrup or sweetener) or yacon syrup

3 tsp orange peel, ground in coffee grinder (*Can also use 1½ tsp alcohol-free orange flavoring,*)

2 Tbsp arrowroot powder

CRUMBLE:

10 Tbsp (about ¾ cup) organic, softened GMO-free Earth Balance[R] spread or organic unrefined sunflower oil or unrefined, virgin coconut oil

1¼ cups gluten-free baking mix

⅛ cup either brown rice syrup, pure maple syrup (unprocessed without added corn syrup or sweetener) or yacon syrup

Pinch of sea or Himalayan salt

1. Preheat oven to 375°F.

2. Combine the rhubarb, berries, ¼ cup sweetener, orange and arrowroot in a bowl. Mix well and transfer to a 13 x 9 baking dish greased with unrefined, virgin coconut oil.

3. In a bowl, combine softened Earth Balance[R] spread or oil, gluten-free flour, ⅛ cup remaining sweetener and salt. The mixture should be well blended and crumbly, but should also stick together.

4. With your hands, sprinkle the flour mixture over the fruit mixture, evenly distributing the mixture over the pan.

5. Bake for about 35-45 minutes, until slightly brown and bubbly.

6. Cool and serve with dairy-free "ice cream" or a dollop of So Delicious® coconut yogurt. You can also add a tablespoon of protein powder for a more fortified breakfast option.

Makes: 8 servings (about 4 cups)
Preparation time: 25 minutes
Baking time: 35 - 45 minutes
Serving size: ½ cup

Corn-Free* | *Nut and Seed-Free* | *Nut or Seed-Free* | *Soy-Free*

* Check labels

HINTS, TIPS AND SUBSTITUTIONS

Can also use crumble from the Apple, Pear or Berry Crisp *on page 222 or from* Date Bars *on page 188.*

If you are sensitive to soy, use the soy-free (red container) version of Earth Balance®.

AMOUNT PER ½ CUP SERVING: Calories 290; Calories from Fat 130; Total Fat 14g; Saturated Fat 6g; Trans Fat 0g; Cholesterol 0mg; Sodium 380mg; Total Carbohydrate 38g; Dietary Fiber 3g; Sugars 10g; Protein 4g; Vitamin A 2%; Vitamin C 80% DV; Calcium 6% DV; Iron 2% DV. *Recipe analyzed with strawberries, brown rice syrup, Earth Balance® spread and sea salt.*

Rhubarb greens and tops are not for human consumption; if you have animals that may eat compost, please discard the tops in the trash.

Smoothies,

Mousse and Pudding

Many of these recipes are pictured on my
website: *www.SweetnessWithoutSugar.com*

*T*hese green smoothie recipes can be modified for your family and children. Smoothies offer a wonderful way to add fresh fruits and vegetables into your diet. Considering that 46% of USDA approved "fruits and vegetables" consumed by kids annually are ketchup and French fries, incorporating even a small portion of smoothie into your child's diet is a step in a healthy direction.

These nutrient-rich smoothies were created with sweetness in mind. If you prefer a smoothie that isn't so sweet, consider using less banana. *Smoothies are at their best when consumed the day they are made.* If you are just beginning this process, try to at least buy organic to replace the conventially-grown produce containing the highest levels of pesticides (as noted in this section and in the chart on page 120).

Read more about the benefits of green smoothies and combining fruit with greens in Victoria Boutenko's book, *Green for Life* (listed in the *Appendix and Resources* section). I hope that you enjoy all of my smoothie recipes, and that you are inspired to try your own combinations and share them with those you love.

When beginning to incorporate green smoothies into your diet, start with small amounts and work toward one quart or more per day. For those of you who regularly enjoy green smoothies or who wish to keep grains separate from fruits and greens, feel free to omit the protein powders. Adding more stevia or other ingredients you desire will help balance the taste (after removing the protein). The recipes here offer a starting point.

As I've noted in earlier sections of the book, I recommend buying organic produce (where possible) because conventionally-grown produce contains pesticides. Select ingredients are noted in the recipes as "organic" because their conventional counterparts would contain the highest levels of pesticides.

ANTIOXIDANT PUNCH SMOOTHIE

Deliciously sweet and power-packed with iron, protein, EFAs and other nutrients, this smoothie can be enjoyed at any time of the day.

1½ frozen bananas

2 small handfuls goji berries (about ⅛ cup)

1 package frozen unsweetened acai berry juice

1 cup frozen organic spinach

1 cup frozen organic strawberries

4 cubes frozen wheatgrass (0.6 oz. each)

3 cups organic unsweetened hemp milk, original flavor

½ cup (2 scoops, or less) Sun Warrior Vanilla Protein[R]

2 Tbsp flax seed oil

1½ cups filtered water

1. In a food processor or blender, use the "high" setting and pureé all ingredients until smooth.

2. Pour into glasses and serve.

Makes: 4 (1½ cup servings)
Preparation time: 10 minutes or less
Serving size: 1½ cups or more

Corn-Free | *Nut and Seed-Free* | *Nut or Seed-Free* | *Soy-Free*

HINTS, TIPS AND SUBSTITUTIONS

Rice milk can be used if you are sensitive to nuts or seeds.

For a raw version of this recipe, please see page 280.

AMOUNT PER 1½ CUP SERVING: Calories 290; Calories from Fat 130; Total Fat 14g; Saturated Fat 1.5g Trans Fat 0g; Cholesterol 0mg; Sodium 160 mg; Total Carbohydrate 23g; Dietary Fiber 5g; Sugars 11g; Protein 15g; Vitamin A 45% DV; Vitamin C 35% DV; Calcium 15% DV; Iron 35% DV. *Recipe analyzed with 2 scoops Sun Warrior Vanilla Protein*[R].

APPLE BLUE SMOOTHIE

Protein, iron, zinc and greens are featured in this nutrient-dense flavorful drink. Bananas contain both B vitamins and potassium.

2 cups filtered water

½ head organic Romaine lettuce

½ organic apple

¼ cup frozen organic blueberries

2 frozen bananas

1 Tbsp black or plain sesame seeds

2 Tbsp pumpkin seeds

¼ cup (1 scoop) Sun Warrior Chocolate Protein® or Nutribiotic®
    Chocolate Rice Protein

½ Tbsp maca powder

½ Tbsp lucuma powder

1. In a food processor or blender, use the "high" setting and pureé all ingredients until smooth.

2. Pour into glasses and serve.

Makes: 4 (1½ cup servings)
Preparation time: 10 minutes or less
Serving size: 1 ½ cups or more

Corn-Free | ~~Nut and Seed-Free~~ | **Nut or Seed-Free** | *Soy-Free*

HINTS, TIPS AND SUBSTITUTIONS

For a raw version of this recipe, please see page 281.

AMOUNT PER 1½ CUP SERVING: Calories 140; Calories from Fat 40; Total Fat 4.5g; Saturated Fat .5g; Trans Fat 0g; Cholesterol 0mg; Sodium 20mg; Total Carbohydrate 22g; Dietary Fiber 3g; Sugars 11g; Protein 7g; Vitamin A 6% DV ; Vitamin C 10% DV; Calcium 2% DV; Iron 10% DV
Recipe analyzed with plain sesame seeds and Sun Warrior Protein®.

BANANA BLUEBERRY SMOOTHIE

Bananas and blueberries always go well together. Strawberries add extra sweetness and vitamin C. This smoothie is easy to digest and has much more flavor than a salad made from seven leaves of lettuce.

This recipe is pictured on the cover.

1 banana

2 cups filtered water

½ cup frozen organic strawberries

½ cup frozen organic blueberries

7 organic Romaine lettuce leaves

¼ cup (1 scoop) Sun Warrior Vanilla Protein[R], ¼ cup (2 scoops) Raw
  Power![TM] Vanilla Protein Superfood Supplement or ¼ cup
  Nutribiotic[R] Vanilla Rice Protein

½ Tbsp maca powder

½ Tbsp lucuma powder

1 Tbsp hempseeds

1 Tbsp flax seed oil or hemp oil

Liquid stevia to taste

1. In a food processor or blender, use the "high" setting and pureé all ingredients until smooth.

2. Pour into glasses and serve.

Makes: 4 (1½ cup servings)
Preparation time: 10 minutes or less
Serving size: 1½ cups or more

Corn-Free | ~~*Nut and Seed-Free*~~ | **Nut or Seed-Free** | *Soy-Free*

HINTS, TIPS AND SUBSTITUTIONS

Brown Rice Protein powder or Raw Power!™ Protein Superfood Supplement also work well in this recipe.

Raw Power!™ Protein Superfood Supplement contains nut protein. Do not use if you are sensitive to nuts.

Omit hempseeds if you are sensitive to seeds.

For a raw version of this recipe, please see page 282.

AMOUNT PER 1½ CUP SERVING: Calories 120; Calories from Fat 45; Total Fat 5g; Saturated Fat 0g; Trans Fat 0g; Cholesterol 0mg; Sodium 20mg; Total Carbohydrate 14g; Dietary Fiber 2g; Sugars 7g; Protein 6g; Vitamin A 6% DV; Vitamin C 20% DV; Calcium 4% DV; Iron 8% DV. *Recipe analyzed with Sun Warrior Protein® and flax oil.*

DIVE INTO YOUR DAY SMOOTHIE

A blend of bittersweet and a hint of ginger. This provides magic for our taste buds, appealing to all of our senses. Chromium, calcium, vitamin K, magnesium and other nutrients are featured in this delicious and unusual smoothie.

2 cups filtered water

½ head of endive

¼ cup (1 scoop) Sun Warrior Chocolate Protein®

⅛ cup (about 2-3 Tbsp) organic pumpkin seeds

1½ cups organic green grapes, stems removed

1 tsp fresh ginger, minced (*If you have a high speed blender, you can use ¼ - ½ inch piece to be minced with the blending.*)

1/16 cup (½ scoop) Raw Power!™ Vanilla Protein Superfood Supplement

½ frozen banana

½ cup unsweetened dairy-free milk (e.g. almond, brown rice or hemp milk)

1 Tbsp acai powder

¼ tsp spirulina powder

1. In a food processor or blender, use the "high" setting and pureé all ingredients until smooth.

2. Pour into glasses and serve.

Makes: 4 (1½ cup servings)
Preparation time: 10 minutes or less
Serving size: 1½ cups or more

Corn-Free | *Nut and Seed-Free* | *Nut or Seed-Free* | *Soy-Free*

HINTS, TIPS AND SUBSTITUTIONS

If you are sensitive to seeds, use rice milk and omit pumpkin seeds.

Raw Power!™ Protein Superfood Supplement contains nut protein. Do not use if you are sensitive to nuts. Substitute with a different protein powder.

For a raw version of this recipe, please see page 284.

AMOUNT PER 1½ CUP SERVING: Calories 160; Calories from Fat 60; Total Fat 7g; Saturated Fat 2g; Trans Fat 0g; Cholesterol 0mg; Sodium 40mg; Total Carbohydrate 20g; Dietary Fiber 4g; Sugars 12g; Protein 8g; Vitamin A 2%; Vitamin C 15% DV; Calcium 8% DV; Iron 10% DV. *Recipe analyzed with: 3 Tbsp pumpkin seeds and Good Karma® rice milk (sweetened with brown rice syrup).*

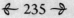

GA GA GOJI COCONUT SMOOTHIE

We often say in our home "gojis make you go go go" and this smoothie will! Though this treat contains just a few ingredients, it's packed with nutrients. May be enjoyed with hemp protein or a sweeter protein powder.

1 organic kale leaf

Large handful goji berries (about ¼ cup)

2 organic celery stalks

4 Tbsp hemp protein powder

1 Tbsp flax seed oil

1 cup coconut water (or add another cup of filtered water)

1 cup filtered water

2 frozen bananas

1. In a food processor or blender, use the "high" setting and pureé all ingredients until smooth.

2. Pour into glasses and serve.

Makes: 4 (1½ cup servings)
Preparation time: 10 minutes or less
Serving size: 1½ cups or more

Corn-Free | *Nut and Seed-Free* | *Nut or Seed-Free* | *Soy-Free*

HINTS, TIPS AND SUBSTITUTIONS

Hemp protein powder gives this smoothie a "greener taste." If you prefer a sweeter taste or are sensitive to seeds, substitute the Nutribiotic[R] *Rice Protein or Raw Power!*™ *Protein Superfood Supplement.*

Raw Power!™ *Protein Superfood Supplement contains nut protein. Do not use if you are sensitive to nuts.*

After blending the smoothie, add stevia if desired.

For a raw version of this recipe, please see page 286.

AMOUNT PER 1½ CUP SERVING: Calories 160; Calories from Fat 40; Total Fat 4.5g; Saturated Fat 0g; Trans Fat 0g; Cholesterol 0mg; Sodium 125mg; Total Carbohydrate 25g; Dietary Fiber 6g; Sugars 14g; Protein 6g; Vitamin A 15%; Vitamin C 25% DV; Calcium 4% DV; Iron 10% DV. *Recipe analyzed with 1 cup coconut water.*

PEACHY KEEN SMOOTHIE

The peaches and bok choy will provide you with extra vitamin C, vitamin A and calcium. Using a variety of fruits and vegetables in your daily smoothies can offer you ways to obtain important nutrients throughout the week.

The Peachy Keen Smoothie pictured on the cover was made without spirulina powder.

2 - 3 cups filtered water

2 bananas (*Frozen bananas give the smoothie a thicker texture and a colder temperature.*)

1 handful (about ¼ cup) organic sunflower seeds

¼ tsp spirulina powder

1 leaf bok choy

¼ tsp lucuma powder

¼ tsp mesquite powder

½ cup (1 scoop) Sun Warrior Natural Protein[R]

1 cup frozen organic peaches

1 Tbsp flax seed oil

1. In a food processor or blender, use the "high" setting and pureé all ingredients until smooth.

2. Pour into glasses and serve.

Makes: 4 (1½ cup servings)
Preparation time: 10 minutes or less
Serving size: 1½ cups or more

Corn-Free | *Nut and Seed-Free* | *Nut or Seed-Free* | *Soy-Free*

HINTS, TIPS AND SUBSTITUTIONS

Omit sunflower seeds if you are sensitive to seeds.

You may substitute Nutribiotic® Rice Protein and add stevia to suit your taste.

For a raw version of this recipe, please see page 287.

AMOUNT PER 1½ CUP SERVING: Calories 160; Calories from Fat 70; Total Fat 8g; Saturated Fat 0.5g; Trans Fat 0g; Cholesterol 0mg; Sodium 40mg; Total Carbohydrate 20g; Dietary Fiber 3g; Sugars 11g; Protein 7g; Vitamin A 6%; Vitamin C 70% DV; Calcium 4% DV; Iron 10% DV. *Recipe analyzed with 2 cups filtered water.*

RAVING RADISHES SMOOTHIE

"Try it, you'll like it" comes to mind here. You may be pleasantly surprised. The ingredients blend well together resulting in a tasty smoothie. This happens to be one of my favorites.

4 radishes

3 beet green leaves

1 cup organic strawberries (can be frozen)

2 frozen bananas

¼ cup (1 scoop) Sun Warrior Chocolate Protein®

1 tsp lucuma powder

1 tsp maca powder

¼ tsp spirulina powder

2 -3 cups filtered water

1 Tbsp flax seed oil or hemp oil

1. In a food processor or blender, use the "high" setting and pureé all ingredients until smooth.

2. Pour into glasses and serve.

Makes: 4 (1½ cup servings)
Preparation time: 10 minutes or less
Serving size: 1½ cups or more

Corn-Free | *Nut and Seed-Free* | *Nut or Seed-Free* | *Soy-Free*

HINTS, TIPS AND SUBSTITUTIONS

You can substitute Nutribiotic® Chocolate Rice Protein or Raw Power!™ Chocolate Protein Superfood Supplement, and add stevia to suit your taste.

Raw Power!™ Protein Superfood Supplement contains nut protein. Do not use if you are sensitive to nuts.

For a raw version of this recipe, please see page 288.

AMOUNT PER 1½ CUP SERVING: Calories 130; Calories from Fat 35; Total Fat 4g; Saturated Fat 0g; Trans Fat 0g; Cholesterol 0mg; Sodium 75mg; Total Carbohydrate 20g; Dietary Fiber 4g; Sugars 10g; Protein 5g; Vitamin A 30%; Vitamin C 60% DV; Calcium 6% DV; Iron 10% DV. *Recipe analyzed with flax seed oil.*

TROPICAL GREEN SMOOTHIE

Here you can eat your peas in smoothie form-providing B vitamins, potassium and calcium. Pineapple contains bromelain, a natural anti-inflammatory enzyme, and manganese, an important trace mineral.

¾ cup frozen pineapple

1½ frozen bananas

Large handful goji berries (about ¼ cup or up to ½ cup)

3 Tbsp unsweetened, unsulphured, shredded organic coconut

1 cup frozen peas

3 cubes frozen wheatgrass (0.6 oz. each)

3 cups organic unsweetened hemp milk, original flavor

½ cup (2 scoops) Sun Warrior Vanilla Protein®

2 Tbsp Nutribiotic® Rice Protein

Filtered water to suit desired texture/consistency

1. In a food processor or blender, use the "high" setting and pureé all ingredients until smooth.

2. Pour into glasses and serve.

Makes: 4 (1½ cup servings)
Preparation time: 10 minutes or less
Serving size: 1½ cups or more

Corn-Free | *Nut and Seed-Free* | *Nut or Seed-Free* | *Soy-Free*

HINTS, TIPS AND SUBSTITUTIONS

You can substitute rice milk if you are sensitive to nuts and seeds.
For a raw version of this recipe, please see page 289.

AMOUNT PER 1½ CUP SERVING: Calories 310; Calories from Fat 80; Total Fat 9g; Saturated Fat 3g; Trans Fat 0g; Cholesterol 0mg; Sodium 170mg; Total Carbohydrate 34g; Dietary Fiber 7g; Sugars 20g; Protein 23g; Vitamin A 2%; Vitamin C 35% DV; Calcium 8% DV; Iron 35% DV. *Recipe analyzed with ½ cup goji berries and ¼ cup filtered water.*

DECADENT CHOCOLATE MOUSSE

Non-tofu fans have eaten this and loved it saying "I can't believe this is tofu!" This is versatile and easy to make. Serve it alone, as a topping, or in the Thumbprint cookies on page 178.

2 (10-oz.) packages of organic silken firm tofu

2 cups unsweetened, dairy-free cocoa

2 Tbsp alcohol-free vanilla flavoring

1 tsp (or up to 3 tsp to suit your taste) alcohol-free orange or berry flavoring

½ cup xylitol (ground in coffee grinder)

⅜ cup maple or coconut sugar crystals (ground in coffee grinder)

Liquid stevia to taste

1. Place all ingredients in a blender and process until smooth.

2. Pour into small bowls and chill for 2 hours or overnight.

3. Serve with strawberries or favorite fruit.

Makes: Approx. 5 cups (serves 8-10)
Preparation time: 15 minutes
Chill time: 2 hours or overnight
Serving size: ½ cup

Corn-Free* | *Nut and Seed-Free* | *Nut or Seed-Free* | *Soy-Free*

* Check labels

HINTS, TIPS AND SUBSTITUTIONS

See the Appendix and Resources *section on page 306 for dairy-free cocoa suggestions.*

This is an alternative way to have a sweet treat and also have protein; a nice "perk" for children (and their parents).

AMOUNT PER ½ CUP SERVING: Calories 130; Calories from Fat 40; Total Fat 4.5g; Saturated Fat 0g; Trans Fat 0g; Cholesterol 0mg; Sodium 0mg; Total Carbohydrate 24g; Dietary Fiber 7g; Sugars 3g; Protein 6g; Calcium 4% DV; Iron 15% DV.

BANANA AVOCADO PUDDING

*Soothing, light, and simple to make. A nice
snack or breakfast side dish.*

This recipe is pictured on the cover (as a smoothie).

¼ cup mashed avocado

2 medium frozen bananas

¼ cup plain So Delicious® coconut yogurt or Ricera® rice yogurt or

   coconut *cream* (not oil)

1. Use a food processor or blender and blend together the banana and avocado.

2. Once the banana and avocado are blended, add "yogurt" and blend to a creamy consistency.

3. Serve right away.

Makes: Approx. 1½ cups
Preparation time: 10 minutes
Serving size: ½ cup

Corn-Free* | *Nut and Seed-Free* | *Nut or Seed-Free* | *Soy-Free*

* Check labels

HINTS, TIPS AND SUBSTITUTIONS

*If you tolerate soy, substitute with a Wildwood Organics™ sprouted
soy yogurt for a higher protein and probiotic content.*

For a raw version of this recipe, please see page 290.

AMOUNT PER ½ CUP SERVING: Calories 110; Calories from Fat 25;
Total Fat 3g; Saturated Fat 1g; Trans Fat 0g; Cholesterol 0mg; Sodium
0mg; Total Carbohydrate 21g; Dietary Fiber 3g; Sugars 11g; Protein
1g; Vitamin A 2% DV; Vitamin C 15% DV; Calcium 4% DV; Iron 2%
DV. *Recipe analyzed with So Delicious® plain coconut yogurt.*

CREAMY FRUIT PUDDING

This dessert blends fruit and fat without elevating blood sugar. Choose your favorite fruits and make an array of delectable creations.

¾ cup favorite fruit (*Peel and core organic apples, organic pears, organic peaches and oranges before blending.*)

2 Tbsp coconut *cream* (not oil)

Filtered water, coconut water or unsweetened, dairy-free milk (e.g. almond, brown rice or hemp milk) to desired consistency

Add liquid stevia to taste

1. Combine all ingredients in a blender and blend until thoroughly mixed.

2. For best results, serve right away. Store additional pudding in the refrigerator. Will keep for 2-3 days in an airtight container.

Makes: Approx. 1½ cups
Preparation time: 10 minutes or less
Serving size: ½ cup

Corn-Free | *Nut and Seed-Free* | *Nut or Seed-Free* | *Soy-Free*

HINTS, TIPS AND SUBSTITUTIONS

For a raw version of this recipe, please see page 291.

For a raw version of this recipe, please see page 291.

AMOUNT PER ½ CUP SERVING: Calories 80; Calories from Fat 35; Total Fat 3.5g; Saturated Fat 3g; Trans Fat 0g; Cholesterol 0mg; Sodium 0mg; Total Carbohydrate 14g; Dietary Fiber 2g; Sugars 7g; Protein 1g; Vitamin C 8% DV; Iron 2% DV. *Recipe analyzed with ¾ cup banana and coconut cream only.*

Raw

and Superfood Treats

Many of these recipes are pictured on my
website: *www.SweetnessWithoutSugar.com*

LAVENDER CHAMOMILE WATER

A nice refreshing and relaxing beverage. Sometimes our sugar cravings indicate a need to slow down and get away from the "to do lists." This is a nice beverage that will help you "take a breather." It can serve as a mini meditation time or break to share alone or with your children. This drink can be steeped for as long as you like, to suit your taste and temperature preferences.

Although not "raw", this drink can be enjoyed by people transitioning into or living a raw food lifestyle.

4 Tbsp organic and/or biodynamically grown lavender

4 cups filtered water

1. Combine lavender and water in a bell jar or glass container. Cover and set in the sun or, during the winter months, in a warm room. *As an alternative, and to save time, try using a French press.*

2. Let this combination sit overnight or up to 24 hours (*less if you prefer a lighter taste*).

3. Pour the lavender water through a tea strainer or colander. Capture the liquid in a pitcher or glass container. Discard the lavender. *If using a French press, push the plunger down, drink the liquid while discarding the lavender.*

4. Drink within 3-4 days. Adjust the amount of lavender to suit your preference.

Makes: 4 cups
Preparation time: 5 minutes
Steeping time: 8 to 24 hours
Serving size: 1 cup

Corn-Free | *Nut and Seed-Free* | *Nut or Seed-Free* | *Soy-Free*

HINTS, TIPS AND SUBSTITUTIONS

You may want to substitute chamomile for lavender. Or, for a nice, calming blend that is great warmed for kids, combine 2 tablespoons lavender with 2 tablespoons chamomile. To make the flavor more subtle, add a little water or sparkling mineral water. If desired, add stevia to taste.

AMOUNT PER 1 CUP SERVING: Calories 5; Calories from Fat 0; Total Fat 0g; Saturated Fat 0g; Trans Fat 0g; Cholesterol 0mg; Sodium 10mg; Total Carbohydrate 1g; Dietary Fiber 0g; Sugars 0g; Protein 0g. *Recipe analyzed with chamomile and filtered spring water.*

SPICED "MILK" (RAW)

Refreshing yet with warming spices, this nice, blended treat provides protein and healthy fat. It's also a soothing, warmed drink before bedtime, on a cold morning or during a cold wintry day.

2 cups raw nut or seed "milk"

¼ tsp cinnamon

¼ tsp cardamom

1-2 Tbsp coconut *cream* (not oil, optional)

12 or less drops of liquid stevia to taste

1. Combine all ingredients and blend to warm briefly or drink as is.

2. Pour into a mug and enjoy.

Makes: 2 cups
Preparation time: 5 - 10 minutes
Serving size: 1 cup

Corn-Free | ~~**Nut and Seed-Free**~~ | **Nut or Seed-Free** | **Soy-Free**

AMOUNT PER 1 CUP SERVING: Calories 330; Calories from Fat 270; Total Fat 30g; Saturated Fat 6g; Trans Fat 0g; Cholesterol 0mg; Sodium 20mg; Total Carbohydrate 11g; Dietary Fiber 6g; Sugars 2g; Protein 11g; Iron 10% DV; Calcium 10% DV. *Recipe analyzed with raw almond milk and 2 Tbsp coconut cream.*

WARMED CHOCOLATE (RAW)

Having met many people with fond memories of drinking hot chocolate during the winter, I've provided this tasty, healthy version for those stormy days when you want to sip it by the fireplace.

1 cup raw nut or seed "milk" (*See recipe on page 256.*)

1 Tbsp, slightly heaping, ground raw cacao

¼ tsp ground cinnamon

1 small vanilla bean, (ground in coffee grinder) or split in half (or ½ tsp
   alcohol-free vanilla flavoring)

Pinch of nutmg and/or cloves or cardamom

4-6 drops liquid stevia (to your taste; can use a flavored stevia if preferred)

1. Combine all ingredients or blend briefly to warm.

2. Serve and enjoy!

Makes: 1 cup
Preparation time: 10 minute
Serving size: 1 cup

Corn-Free | ~~Nut and Seed-Free~~ | *Nut or Seed-Free* | *Soy-Free*

Amount per 1 cup serving: Calories 330; Calories from Fat 230; Total
Fat 25g; Saturated Fat 2g; Trans Fat 0g; Cholesterol 0mg; Sodium 20mg;
Total Carbohydrate 11g; Dietary Fiber 5g; Sugars 10g; Protein 12g;
Calcium 10% DV; Iron 10% DV *Recipe analyzed with raw, unsweetened
almond milk using a ratio of 2 cups almonds to 6 cups filtered water.*

SPARKLING WATER WITH STEVIA FLAVORS

Since 1978, consumption of soft drinks has more than tripled for boys and doubled for girls. My sparkling drink is a great alternative to soda! With this recipe, you can still enjoy the "bubbles" and sweet flavors reminiscent of soda. There are so many stevia flavors to choose from such as root beer, grape, orange and more. Adding apple juice to sparkling water brings back memories of a trip to England where "appletizers" (a very sweet, carbonated apple drink), were offered in most restaurants.

Although not "raw", this drink can be enjoyed by people transitioning into or living a raw food lifestyle.

8 oz. Gerlosteiner[R] or other sparkling water

Add one of the following:

4 or more drops of flavored stevia

1 orange 1 apple, or ½ grapefruit (fresh-squeezed)

1. Combine Gerlosteiner[R] or mineral water with one of the flavorings listed above.

2. Mix well and enjoy. *For extra fun, drink with a straw.*

Makes: 1 cup
Preparation time: 5 minutes
Serving size: 1 cup

Corn-Free | *Nut and Seed-Free* | *Nut or Seed-Free* | *Soy-Free*

SPARKLING WATER WITH STEVIA FLAVORS:

AMOUNT PER SERVING: Calories 0; Calories from Fat 0; Total Fat 0g; Saturated Fat 0g; Trans Fat 0 g; Cholesterol 0 mg; Sodium 30mg; Total Carbohydrate 0g; Dietary Fiber 0g; Sugars 0g; Protein 0g; Calcium 8% DV. *Recipe analyzed with stevia and Gerlosteiner® water.*

SPARKLING WATER WITH 2 OZ. FRESH-SQUEEZED ORANGE JUICE:

AMOUNT PER SERVING: Calories 30; Calories from Fat 0; Total Fat 0g; Saturated Fat 0g; Trans Fat 0g; Cholesterol 0mg; Sodium 30mg; Total Carbohydrate 6g; Dietary Fiber 0g; Sugars 5g; Protein 0g; Vitamin A 2% DV; Vitamin C 50% DV; Calcium 8% DV. *Recipe analyzed with ¼ cup fresh-squeezed orange juice and Gerlosteiner® water.*

COCONUT KEFIR

Making this drink is worth the effort. Once the coconuts are opened, the rest is easy. Kefir is wonderful for helping to restore gut health and for minimizing sugar and sweet cravings. It will also offer a healthy bacteria perk when you're travelling or in the midst of cold and flu season.

Although not "RAW", this drink can be enjoyed by people transitioning into or living a raw food lifestyle.

3-4 Thai young coconuts (the white cone-shaped coconuts)

1 packet kefir culture (the Body Ecology® brand works very well)

1. Using a sharp knife, cut slices from the bottom of the coconuts (the flat side) until you see the brown or white ring/soft spot.

2. Using an apple corer, vegetable peeler or small paring knife, poke a hole in the soft spot (the round ring) near or at the location of the brown or white spot. Use a peeler to dig the hole out.

3. Prepare to overturn the coconut and capture the liquid in a measuring cup or glass bell jar. Drain. Set the coconut water aside after making sure it is a light tan/yellow color. Coconut water that is pink in color should be discarded. Repeat these steps with each coconut until you collect one quart of liquid.

4. Add kefir starter culture (purchased from a health food store or online via the link noted under "Hints" on the next page).

5. Cover the quart of liquid and shake it well. For best results, place in a warm room for 2-3 days. Kefir will be ready when small bubbles appear after the container is moved slightly.

6. Enjoy this bubbly, refreshing and healthy drink. If giving kefir to children, start with 1-2 ounces at a time and work up from there to ½ cup.

Makes: 1 quart (4 cups)
Preparation time: 30 minutes or more
Waiting time: 3 days
Serving size: 1 oz. for babies/ ½ cup or more for toddlers/
1 cup for adults

Corn-Free | *Nut and Seed-Free* | *Nut or Seed-Free* | *Soy-Free*

HINTS, TIPS AND SUBSTITUTIONS

To view a description and demonstration of how to make this delicious and healthy drink, visit

www.bodyecology.com/mcoconutkefir.php.

I recommend reviewing this site for details on how to prepare the liquid and scoop out the fresh coconut! Yum! We have had positive results using one packet of kefir culture for two Thai coconuts (without straining or heating beforehand) though the quantity of liquid is less than a full quart.

If you have a strong sensitivity to sugar (e.g. candida, sugar addictions, etc.), you may wish to increase your serving size initially (on an individual basis) or contact me for a consultation.

AMOUNT PER 1 CUP SERVING: Calories 40; Calories from Fat 5; Total Fat .5g; Saturated Fat 0g; Trans Fat 0g; Cholesterol 0mg; Sodium 220mg; Total Carbohydrate 8g; Dietary Fiber 2g; Sugars 6g; Protein 2g; Vitamin C 8% DV; Calcium 4% DV; Iron 4% DV.

When our children were seven months old, we gave them one ounce of kefir per day (as a test, for 3-4 days). Their bodies handled it well and they seemed to love the drink! Our son, Solomon enjoys a 4-6 ounce serving of kefir whenever his immune system needs a little boost.

HOMEMADE NUT OR SEED "MILK" (RAW)

This easy "milk" recipe was inspired by drinks featured in Laura Bruno's <u>The Lazy Raw Foodist's Guide</u>. Laura's wonderful resource guide (which is for everyone, even non-raw foodists) includes tips and recipe variations. When using the Jack LaLanne Power Elite Juicer®, this "milk" is simple to make!

2 cups raw, soaked nuts or seeds

3-6 cups filtered water

2 pitted dates (optional)

Liquid stevia to taste

1. Soak the nuts or seeds in filtered water. (See the chart on page 134 for more information on soaking and sprouting times for nuts and seeds.) Drain.

2. Blend soaked nuts or seeds with new filtered water. Use enough water to create your desired thickness. *Combining three or four parts water to one part nuts will create "milk" most people enjoy. For example, use 1 cup nuts to 3-4 cups of filtered water.*

3. If desired, drink the milk plain. You can also sweeten the milk with enough drops of stevia to suit your taste, or add pitted dates and re-blend.

4. Set aside a big bowl and a sprout bag or cheesecloth. *(Cheesecloth is messier to use.)* Pour the liquid into a sprout bag and drain into bowl. Squeeze the contents to get more liquid out of the "pulp." For a pictorial demonstration of raw nut or milk preparation, visit this link: *www.rawglow.com/ almondmilkhowto.htm.*

Makes: 3 to 6 cups "milk"
Soaking time: varies 2-12 hours
Blend and strain time: 20 minutes
Serving size: ½ cup toddler, 1 cup adult

Corn-Free | ~~*Nut and Seed-Free*~~ | **Nut or Seed-Free** | *Soy-Free*

HINTS, TIPS AND SUBSTITUTIONS

Use the chart on page 134 to determine soaking time. If soaking time is between 8-12 hours, soaking the nuts/seeds overnight is easiest.

AMOUNT PER 1 CUP SERVING: Calories 300; Calories from Fat 210; Total Fat 24g; Saturated Fat 2g; Trans Fat 0g; Cholesterol 0mg; Sodium 5mg; Total Carbohydrate 16g; Dietary Fiber 6g; Sugars 7g; Protein 10g; Calcium 15% DV; Iron 10% DV. *Recipe analyzed with 2 cups raw almonds, 2 dates and 6 cups filtered water.*

NUT BALLS (RAW)

This recipe, inspired by Dr. Joseph Mercola, was once referred to as halvah. But when a dear friend repeatedly asked me to bring "those nut balls" to our get-togethers, the "nut ball" name stuck. Since then, many new versions of nut balls have emerged. All freeze well and can stay in the refrigerator for up to two weeks in an airtight container (if they aren't gobbled up before then!)

½ cup ground raw walnuts, almonds, cashews or pecans, (ground in coffee grinder or blender with a dry blade attachment) or use dehydrated meal flours leftover from nut milks (almond meal or hazelnut meal)

½ cup dehydrated coconut "meat" from a Thai young coconut, shredded

½ cup (4 scoops) hemp protein or ½ cup (4 scoops) Raw Power!™ Protein Superfood Supplement, or ¾ cup (1½ scoops) Sun Warrior Natural or Vanilla Protein[R]

½ cup raw unsalted and unsweetened almond, cashew or sesame butter (e.g. almond butter or tahini)

¼ cup raw coconut water/milk (*Can also blend inner "meat" of young Thai coconut. Use more or less to suit your taste and consistency preferences.*)

½ cup dehydrated blueberries, or other berry of choice

6-10 Tbsp yacon syrup or Jerusalem artichoke syrup or 5 drops liquid stevia (or to taste)

1. Combine all ingredients in a bowl. Can use a coffee grinder or a dry blade to grind nuts into a fine powder.

2. Use a spoon to mix until the combination stays together. (*Add more coconut water/milk to suit your taste and texture preferences.*)

3. Scoop into balls using a heaping teaspoon.

4. These can be served immediately or stored in the refrigerator (if they aren't eaten before they get to the refrigerator). If desired, sprinkle with dried coconut or raw cacao. These also store well in the freezer.

Makes: 32 balls
Preparation time: 15 minutes
Serving size: 2 balls

Corn-Free | ~~*Nut and Seed-Free*~~ | *Nut or Seed-Free* | *Soy-Free*

HINTS, TIPS AND SUBSTITUTIONS

If you are sensitive to nuts, try sunflower or pumpkin seeds.

For those needing extra sweetness, add a drop of stevia to the outside of the ball before eating. Coat it with your fingers to evenly distribute the sweet flavor.

Consider doubling this recipe. They'll go fast!

AMOUNT PER 2 BALL SERVING: Calories 230; Calories from Fat 80; Total Fat 9g; Saturated Fat 2.5g; Trans Fat 0g; Cholesterol 0mg; Sodium 10mg; Total Carbohydrate 11g; Dietary Fiber 5g; Sugars 4g; Protein 4g; Vitamin C 10% DV; Calcium 4% DV; Iron 4% DV. *Recipe analyzed using raw pecans, raw tahini, Sun Warrior Natural Protein*[R], *fresh coconut water, dried blueberries and 8 Tbsp yacon syrup.*

These healthy treats contain omega fats, protein and other nutrients, and always provide sweet smiles. One serving is quite satisfying.

TAHINI ORANGE TURKISH TAFFY (RAW)

Here is a way to have taffy without it sticking to your teeth. The delicious flavor continues to unfold in your mouth. It is also packed with protein and fiber.

½ cup raw unsalted and unsweetened tahini

¾ cup packed chopped soaked dates (when chopped and pressed down, they measure ¾c)

½ cup water from soaked dates

2 tsp minced fresh ginger

2 tsp orange peel (zest)

1 tsp alcohol-free orange flavoring

½ cup (2 scoops) Sun Warrior Natural Protein[R]

5-9 tsp psyllium husk powder

Liquid stevia to taste

1. Blend tahini, soaked dates and water, ginger, orange peel, orange flavor and protein powder in a Cuisinart[R] or blender.

2. Gradually add up to five teaspoons of psyllium husk (one teaspoon at a time) and blend after each addition, until mixture is smooth, but firm enough to form into balls.

3. Let the mixture sit for up to 15 minutes. If necessary, add more psyllium. Psyllium takes a little time to fully absorb.

4. Use a teaspoon to form into balls. Chill taffy balls in the refrigerator or freezer.

Makes: Approx. 20 pieces
Preparation time: 20 minutes
Serving size: 2 pieces

Corn-Free | ~~*Nut and Seed-Free*~~ | *Nut or Seed-Free* | *Soy-Free*

HINTS, TIPS AND SUBSTITUTIONS

You can also replace the Sun Warrior Natural Protein® with Raw Power!™ Protein Superfood Supplement Original or Vanilla Flavor, and add more stevia to the finished taffy for extra flavor.

Raw Power!™ Protein Superfood Supplement® contains nuts. Substitute this ingredient with a different protein powder if making a nut-free version of this recipe.

AMOUNT PER 2 PIECE SERVING: Calories 130; Calories from Fat 70; Total Fat 8g; Saturated Fat 1g; Trans Fat 0g; Cholesterol 0mg; Sodium 10mg; Total Carbohydrate 15g; Dietary Fiber 3g; Sugars 8g; Protein 6g; Vitamin C 2% DV; Calcium 8% DV; Iron 8%DV. *Recipe analyzed with nine teaspoons psyllium husk powder.*

GOJI GO BON BONS (RAW)

These provide high-quality protein, absorbable greens, fiber and antioxidants. They are easy to take with you for travel, lunches, snacks and picnics. Even those who aren't fans of the goji taste will enjoy the subtle flavors of this healthy bon bon. If you like the taste of spirulina, adding more in this recipe works well.

1 cup raw unsalted and unsweetened almond or hempseed butter

⅛ cup (½ scoop) Sun Warrior Protein[R], any flavor

⅛ cup or 2 Tbsp hemp protein powder

¼ cup ground goji berries (ground in coffee grinder)

½ tsp spirulina powder

1 tsp acai powder

¼ cup ground flax seed (ground in coffee grinder)

¼ cup yacon syrup or Jerusalem artichoke syrup or liquid stevia to taste

For rolling or outer coating:

Ground goji berries

Hempseeds

Shredded dehydrated organic coconut flakes

Raw cacao nibs (whole or ground in coffee grinder - to your preference)

1. Combine all ingredients in a medium-sized bowl.

2. Use your hands to shape the mixture into teaspoon-sized balls.

3. Roll balls to coat them in any of the above options or eat as is.

4. Store in an airtight container in the refrigerator until ready to eat.

Makes: 30 bon bons
Preparation time: 20 minutes
Serving size: 2 bon bons

Corn-Free | ~~*Nut and Seed-Free*~~ | *Nut or Seed-Free* | *Soy-Free*

HINTS, TIPS AND SUBSTITUTIONS

Check manufacturer information to learn if these sweeteners are raw for your raw diet. If not, soaked dates or figs can be blended and added to suit your desired taste.

AMOUNT PER 2 BON BON SERVING WITHOUT OUTER COATING: Calories 170; Calories from Fat 60; Total Fat 7g; Saturated Fat .5g; Trans Fat 0g; Cholesterol 0mg; Sodium 15mg; Total Carbohydrate 9g; Dietary Fiber 3g; Sugars 3g; Protein 8g; Vitamin C 6% DV; Iron 15% DV *Recipe analyzed with hempseed butter and yacon syrup.*

NUTTY CRUNCH BON BONS (RAW)

I like these for their flavor and crunch. They have a nice blend of essential fatty acids and protein. They are also easy and fun to make with a child. Eating "the batter" when it sticks to your hands can create laughter and great memories for everyone involved.

⅔ cup raw, unsalted and unsweetened, hempseed butter, pumpkin seed butter or Brazil nut butter

⅔ cup raw, unsalted and unsweetened, cashew or almond butter

⅛ cup yacon or Jerusalem artichoke syrup or 5-10 drops liquid stevia (or to suit your taste)

⅛ tsp sea or Himalayan salt

2 tsp alcohol-free vanilla flavoring or other flavoring (or equivalent quantity of ground vanilla bean to suit your taste)

1½ cup raw granola cereal

1. Combine nut butters, sweetener, salt and vanilla and mix together well with a spoon or your hands.

2. Add raw cereal of choice and fold into the mixture.

3. With your hands (or your child's), form teaspoon-sized balls. You can also make bars by spreading mixture evenly into the bottom of an 8 x 8 pan.

Makes: 24 bon bons or bars
Preparation time: 15 minutes
Serving size: 2 bon bons or bars

Corn-Free* | ~~Nut and Seed-Free~~ | **Nut or Seed-Free** | **Soy-Free**

* Check labels

HINTS, TIPS AND SUBSTITUTIONS

Varying the nut or seed butters will provide different nutrients. If sensitive to nuts, use seed butter only.

Some may prefer more sweetener, depending upon taste and nut butter used.

Dip bon bons into Raw Chocolate Topping (on page 270) or drizzle sauce on top of bon bons. If you are using the pan, you can "make a picture" by drizzling the chocolate sauce onto the top of the bars.

AMOUNT PER 2 BON BON SERVING: Calories 270; Calories from Fat 130; Total Fat 14g; Saturated Fat 1.5g; Trans Fat 0g; Cholesterol 0mg; Sodium 20mg; Total Carbohydrate 16g; Dietary Fiber 5g; Sugars 2g; Protein 11g; Vitamin C 4% DV ; Calcium 4% DV; Iron 20% DV. *Recipe analyzed with raw hempseed and almond butters, yacon and Lydia's Organic™ Sprouted Cinnamon Cereal and without a chocolate topping.*

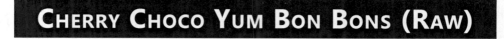

CHERRY CHOCO YUM BON BONS (RAW)

These are full of flavor, essential fatty acids, and fiber.
They also have a pretty pinkish-purple hue.

This recipe is pictured on the cover.

½ cup raw chia seeds

½ cup raw sesame seeds

½ cup raw sunflower seeds

1 cup dehydrated coconut "meat" from a Thai young coconut, shredded
  or finely ground

1 cup frozen or dehydrated cherries (*If frozen, drain them once thawed.*)

1 cup golden raisins (*Mulberries are also delicious in this recipe.*)

½ cup (2 scoops) Sun Warrior Chocolate Protein[R]

¼ cup (1 scoop) Sun Warrior Vanilla Protein[R]

1 cup raw unsalted and unsweetened tahini

¼ plus ⅛ cup raw coconut water

Variations:

Dates, figs, apricots, goji berries or other dried fruits may
  replace cherries or raisins. Unsulphured, unsweetened
  varieties are best.

Replace tahini with nut butters (almond, cashew, pistachio, Brazil
  nut, etc.).

Replace nuts with seeds.

1. In a Cuisinart® or blender, grind seeds, coconut, cherries, and raisins until ground into a moist and gooey consistency.

2. Into the food processor or blender, add the gooey mixture, ¼ cup of the chocolate protein powder and ¼ cup of vanilla powder. Process or blend until the mixture becomes thick. Transfer this mixture into a large mixing bowl. Add the remaining amount of protein powder and mix by hand. Add tahini and coconut water, and mix until the ingredients stay together well. Add liquid stevia to suit your taste.

3. Use a teaspoon to form mixture into balls, or press mixture into an 8" pan. Chill in refrigerator or freezer.

Makes: Approx. 24 bon bons
Preparation time: 15 minutes
Serving size: 2 bon bons

Corn-Free | *Nut and Seed-Free* | **Nut or Seed-Free** | *Soy-Free*

AMOUNT PER 2 BON BON SERVING: Calories 340; Calories from Fat 200; Total Fat 22g; Saturated Fat 7g; Trans Fat 0g; Cholesterol 0mg; Sodium 30mg; Total Carbohydrate 23g; Dietary Fiber 5g; Sugars 12g; Protein 12g; Vitamin A 2% DV; Vitamin C 2% DV; Calcium 15% DV; Iron 20% DV. *Recipe analyzed with frozen cherries and golden raisins.*

You can also make this recipe in bar form by pressing the mixture into an 8-inch round dish before slicing.

MOLASSES "MMM" TRUFFLES (RAW)

These have the distinctive taste of molasses. Vitamin C-packed camu camu and iron-rich molasses give this tasty truffle an added boost.

1 cup raw, unsalted, unsweetened nut and seed blend (either purchased
  pre-made, or prepared by hand (e.g. ½ cup raw almond butter
  plus ½ cup raw sunflower seed butter))

½ cup rice bran

2 tsp maca powder

2 Tbsp molasses or yacon syrup or Jerusalem artichoke syrup

1½ tsp yacon syrup

½ tsp camu camu powder

⅛ cup (1 scoop) Raw Power!™ Protein Superfood Supplement

1 Tbsp raw coconut *cream* (not oil)

1 dropper lemon stevia

2 Tbsp hempseeds

3 Tbsp dehydrated blueberries (unsweetened, corn syrup and sugar-free)

2 Tbsp dehydrated cherries (unsweetened, corn syrup and sugar-free)

1 tsp alcohol-free vanilla flavoring or vanilla bean powder

½ tsp raw cacao powder

2 dashes of cinnamon

1. Combine all ingredients in a medium bowl. Mix together with your hands or
   a spoon.

2. Use a teaspoon to form into truffle balls. Serve or store.

Makes: Approx. 24 truffles
Preparation time: 15 minutes
Serving size: 2 truffles

Corn-Free | ~~*Nut and Seed-Free*~~ | *Nut or Seed-Free* | *Soy-Free*

HINTS, TIPS AND SUBSTITUTIONS

If sensitive to nuts, use seed butter only.

Raw Power!™ Protein Superfood Supplement® contains nuts. Substitute this ingredient with a different protein powder if making a nut-free version of this recipe.

Liquid vanilla flavoring is often more concentrated than vanilla bean powder, so it imparts a stronger flavor in a smaller quantity than vanilla bean powder. If choosing vanilla bean powder, you may wish to use more than 1 tsp to create the flavor you like.

AMOUNT PER 2 TRUFFLE SERVING: Calories 220; Calories from Fat 100; Total Fat 11g; Saturated Fat 1.5g; Trans Fat 0g; Cholesterol 0mg; Sodium 5mg; Total Carbohydrate 13g; Dietary Fiber 5g; Sugars 3g; Protein 8g; Vitamin C 6% DV; Calcium 4% DV; Iron 15% DV. *Recipe analyzed with ½ cup raw almond butter, ½ cup raw hempseed butter and yacon instead of molasses. The sweetener change will alter the flavor. If you follow a raw lifestyle and are open to using molasses, I suggest you use it. Molasses gives these truffles a unique and distinct flavor.*

Check manufacturer information to learn if these sweeteners are raw for your raw diet. If not, soaked dates or figs can be blended and added to suit your desired taste. Molasses is not considered a raw sweetener; both yacon and Jerusalem artichoke syrup have rich flavors.

RAW CHOCOLATE TOPPING

If you are a chocolate lover, it is hard to create a bad chocolate sauce. Truth be told, even if a dessert doesn't taste as good as you had hoped, adding a little bit of chocolate topping "makes it all better." Delicious plain or on a bon bon.

½ cup raw cacao powder

Liquid stevia to suit your sweet taste

¼ cup (or more) of raw coconut water

1 vanilla bean, ground (*Add more vanilla bean to suit your taste.*)

1. Using a spoon, combine ingredients to create a topping with your desired consistency.

2. Spread or drizzle topping over your favorite dessert.

Makes: ½ cup or more (depending upon amt of liquid used)
Preparation time: 5 minutes
Serving size: ⅛ cup or 2 Tbsp

Corn-Free | Nut and Seed-Free | Nut or Seed-Free | Soy-Free

HINTS, TIPS AND SUBSTITUTIONS

This recipe can be prepared by replacing the raw cacao with ½ cup raw carob.

Using lucuma powder plus yacon syrup (to your taste) also creates a delicious topping.

AMOUNT PER 2 TBSP SERVING: Calories 90; Calories from Fat 15; Total Fat 1.5g; Saturated Fat 0g; Trans Fat 0g; Cholesterol 0mg; Sodium 30mg; Total Carbohydrate 1g; Dietary Fiber 0g; Sugars 14g; Protein 4g; Vitamin C 2% DV. *Recipe analyzed with ½ cup fresh coconut water.*

RAW FUDGE

*This recipe was inspired by other delicious raw fudge recipes.
It can be prepared with raw carob or raw chocolate. Many people
have asked for this recipe and are amazed that the sweet taste
comes only from fruits and the hint of coconut oil.*

¾ cup unrefined, virgin, raw coconut oil, warmed until liquid (measure
      ¾ cup of melted oil)

1 cup pitted soft dates

½ cup mulberries, raisins, currants, dehydrated cherries or goji berries

1 tsp maca powder (optional; adds more superfood nutrition)

Dash of cinnamon

1 tsp alcohol-free vanilla flavoring or vanilla bean powder

¼ cup raw carob powder

¼ cup raw cacao powder

¼ cup extra raw carob or raw cacao powder

⅓ cup (about 2 scoops) Sun Warrior Protein[R] or (about 4 scoops) Raw
      Power![TM] Protein Superfood Supplement

1½ cups raw walnuts, soaked 2 hours, then drained and dried (still
      yummy without these too)

1. In a small saucepan over very low heat, melt the coconut oil and measure to
    ¾ cup. *Coconut oil will melt in a heated room. If the oil is solid, spoon it from
    the jar into a saucepan and allow it to melt without reaching high-heat. This
    will preserve the nutrients in the oil.* Use a food processor to blend the dates,
    berries of choice and coconut oil. Process until smooth.

2. Add maca (if using), cinnamon, vanilla, raw chocolate (or carob), and protein
    powder and process again.

3. Transfer the mixture from a food processor into a bowl and add the walnuts
    (if using).

4. Knead the walnuts into the mixture. Pack the fudge firmly into an 8 x 8 pan. Fudge should be approximately one-inch thick. Slice into 16 pieces.

5. Refrigerate for an hour prior to serving. Fudge stored in a closed container in the refrigerator will last up to one month.

Makes: 16 pieces
Preparation time: 25 minutes
Serving size: 1 piece

Corn-Free | *Nut and Seed-Free* | *Nut or Seed-Free* | *Soy-Free*

HINTS, TIPS AND SUBSTITUTIONS

Preparing this fudge in steps, as noted above, makes a difference since it is a thick mixture. Though I often just put things together and blend, for this recipe, I recommend following the instructions.

Liquid vanilla flavoring is often more concentrated than vanilla bean powder, so it imparts a stronger flavor in a smaller quantity than vanilla bean powder. If choosing vanilla bean powder, you may wish to use more than 1 tsp to create the flavor you like.

This recipe can be prepared by replacing the ¼ cup carob, ¼ cup carob or cacao, with 1) ¾ cup raw carob only, or 2) ¾ cup raw cacao only.

The fruits and superfoods in this fudge contain beneficial nutrients. The fudge is also made with cacao/chocolate, which affects people differently. My recommendation is to listen to your body when determining your optimum serving size.

AMOUNT PER 1 PIECE SERVING: Calories 220; Calories from Fat 130; Total Fat 15g; Saturated Fat 7g; Trans Fat 0g; Cholesterol 0mg; Sodium 10mg; Total Carbohydrate 16g; Dietary Fiber 2g; Sugars 15g; Protein 6g; Vitamin C 15% DV; Calcium 4% DV; Iron 6% DV. *Recipe analyzed with mulberries, ¾ cup raw cacao, Sun Warrior Protein® and walnuts.*

EASY FROZEN FRUIT TREAT

You may use fresh-squeezed juices from your favorite fruits (apple, mango, pear, pineapple, orange, etc.). This is a good recipe for people who are transitioning away from refined sugar and also craving a sweet treat. They are easy to make, easy to grab from the freezer and are free of dyes, unhealthy sweeteners and chemicals. The added oil helps to balance your blood sugar. These frozen treats also bring relief to teething babies.

Although not "raw", this treat can be enjoyed by people transitioning into or living a raw food lifestyle.

FOR 8 (½ cup size) FROZEN TREATS (2 servings of fruit per treat):

4 cups fresh-squeezed juice

2 tsp flax seed oil or hemp oil

Add liquid stevia to taste before freezing. (*Do not use powdered stevia for this recipe.*)

FOR 1 (½ cup sixze) FROZEN TREAT (2 servings of fruit for a toddler):

½ cup fresh-squeezed juice

¼ tsp flax seed oil or hemp oil

Add liquid stevia to taste before freezing. (*Do not use powdered stevia for this recipe.*)

FOR 1 (¼ cup size) FROZEN TREAT (1 serving of fruit for a toddler):

¼ cup fresh-squeezed juice

¼ cup filtered water

¼ tsp flax seed oil or hemp oil

Add liquid stevia to taste before freezing. (*Do not use powdered stevia for this recipe.*)

1. Using a blender, combine ingredients to help emulsify the oil.

2. Add liquid stevia to taste. Re-blend.

3. Pour contents into ice pop molds and freeze for four hours or more.

Makes: 8 standard-size frozen treats (using ice pop molds)
Preparation time: 10 minutes or less
Freezing time: 4 hours or more
Serving size: 1 frozen treat

Corn-Free | *Nut and Seed-Free* | *Nut or Seed-Free* | *Soy-Free*

HINTS, TIPS AND SUBSTITUTIONS

The "standard size" single treat holds a half cup of liquid. These are the size of a push-pop or half the size of a "wide" Fudgsicle®. These molds are often sold in sets of four. This recipe will prepare enough frozen treats for two sets.

If sensitive to nuts and seeds, substitute with a different oil.

If trying these treats with your teething baby, I suggest using a fruit your child has handled well and enjoyed.

AMOUNT PER 1 (½ CUP) ICE POP SERVING (2 FRUIT PER SERVING VERSION):
Calories 70; Calories from Fat 15; Total Fat 1.5g; Saturated Fat 0g; Trans Fat 0g; Cholesterol 0mg; Sodium 0mg; Total Carbohydrate 13g; Dietary Fiber 0g; Sugars 10g; Protein 1g; Vitamin A 4% DV; Vitamin C 100% DV; Calcium 2% DV; Iron 2% DV. *Recipe analyzed with fresh-squeezed orange juice and flax oil.*

FRUITY FROZEN YOGURT

This recipe is wonderful for vegans (and non-vegans) who seek delicious alternatives to ice cream, Popsicles® and frozen yogurt. This can also be eaten instantly, like a smoothie, or as a topping over cereal.

Although not "raw", this treat can be enjoyed by people transitioning into or living a raw food lifestyle.

2 cups organic raspberries or blueberries

1½ Tbsp fresh lemon juice

Liquid stevia to taste

½ cup raw coconut pulp (*Add more to suit your taste and desired consistency.*)

½ cup raw coconut water

¼ cup raw coconut *cream* (not oil)

1. Pureé raspberries and lemon juice. If desired, strain out the seeds using a fine mesh strainer.

2. Add liquid stevia to taste.

3. Blend raspberries and lemon with the rest of the ingredients.

4. Pour into a freezer-safe container or into ice pop molds. If you want a creamier texture, thaw the mixture until soft, but not thoroughly melted, then re-blend the mixture. Refreeze the second blending and serve when ready to eat.

Makes: 2 cups (about 4 standard-size ice pops)
Preparation time: 10 minutes or less
Freezing time: 4 hours or more
Serving size: ½ cup or 1 ice pop

Corn-Free | *Nut and Seed-Free* | *Nut or Seed-Free* | *Soy-Free*

HINTS, TIPS AND SUBSTITUTIONS

Raspberries (especially frozen ones) can be tart. More stevia may be needed to suit your taste.

AMOUNT PER ½ CUP SERVING OR 1 ICE POP: Calories 180; Calories from Fat 140; Total Fat 16g; Saturated Fat 14g; Trans Fat 0g; Cholesterol 0mg; Sodium 35mg; Total Carbohydrate 13g; Dietary Fiber 1g; Sugars 1g; Protein 2g; Vitamin C 30%; Calcium 2% DV; Iron 8% DV. *Recipe analyzed with raspberries.*

CREAMY ORANGE ICE POP (RAW)

Enjoy this frozen confection reminiscent of the "oldie but goodie". This version contains fiber, Vitamin C, protein, fat and sugar from fresh oranges only! This can be part of a meal from a parents' point of view and a treat from a kids' perspective. Everybody's happy.

2 seedless oranges, peeled and de-seeded

1 cup raw coconut meat

¼ cup plus ⅛ cup of freshly-squeezed orange juice (juice from 1
   medium orange)

5 Tbsp coconut *cream* (not oil)

5 tsp alcohol-free vanilla flavoring

12-15 drops SteviaClear[R] Vanilla Crème flavor (*Add more to suit your taste.*)

1. In a blender, blend together all ingredients (on high) until smooth. If desired, blend for less time to retain the "pulpy" texture.

2. Pour into the ice pop molds or ice cube trays. Freeze for 4 hours or more. *Fills approximately 1 ¼ ice cube trays.*

Makes: 6 thin ½ cup molded ice pops
Preparation time: 10 minutes or less
Freezing time: 4 hours or more
Serving size: 1 ice pop or 3 cubes

Corn-Free | Nut and Seed-Free | Nut or Seed-Free | Soy-Free

AMOUNT PER 1 (½ CUP) ICE POP SERVING: Calories 210; Calories from Fat 160; Total Fat 18g; Saturated Fat 16g; Trans Fat 0g; Cholesterol 0mg; Sodium 0mg; Total Carbohydrate 11g; Dietary Fiber 2g; Sugars 6g; Protein 2g; Vitamin A 2% DV; Vitamin C 50% DV; Calcium 2% DV; Iron 8% DV. *Recipe analyzed with fresh coconut meat/cream.*

RAW "MILK" SHAKE

This is so easy to make! It tastes like a regular milkshake and contains protein! When flavoring with chocolate or vanilla protein powder, you can't go wrong. Great for kids of all ages.

1 cup raw nut or raw seed milk (*See chart on page 134 for soaking suggestions.*)

2-3 bananas, frozen

2 cups filtered water

Chocolate- or vanilla-flavored protein powder (choose one):

    ⅛ cup (1 scoop) Raw Power!™ Protein Superfood Supplement®, or

    ¼ cup (1 scoop) Sun Warrior Protein®

1. Combine ingredients in a blender until smooth. Add enough liquid to create your preferred consistency.

2. Pour into a glass, serve and enjoy.

Makes: 4 cups
Preparation time: 10 minutes
Serving size: 1 cup

Corn-Free | Nut and Seed-Free | Nut or Seed-Free | Soy-Free

HINTS, TIPS AND SUBSTITUTIONS

For more protein, add more powder to your glass or drink more than one cup. It's easy!

Raw Power!™ Protein Superfood Supplement® contains nuts. Substitute a different protein powder if making a nut-free version of this recipe.

AMOUNT PER 1 CUP SERVING: Calories 170; Calories from Fat 60; Total Fat 7g; Saturated Fat .5g; Trans Fat 0g; Cholesterol 0mg; Sodium 20mg; Total Carbohydrate 23g; Dietary Fiber 4g; Sugars 11g; Protein 8g; Vitamin A 2% DV; Vitamin C 15% DV; Calcium 6% DV; Iron 8% DV. *Recipe analyzed using raw almond milk without dates, 3 bananas and Sun Warrior Natural Protein Powder®.*

ANTIOXIDANT PUNCH SMOOTHIE (RAW)

Deliciously sweet and power-packed with iron, protein, EFAs and other nutrients, this smoothie can be enjoyed at any time of the day.

1½ frozen bananas

2 small handfuls goji berries (about ⅛ cup)

1 package frozen unsweetened acai berry juice

1 cup frozen organic spinach

1 cup frozen organic strawberries

4 cubes frozen wheatgrass (0.6 oz. each)

2 cups raw nut or seed milk (*See page 256 for recipe basics.*)

½ cup (2 scoops, or less) Sun Warrior Vanilla Protein[R]

2 Tbsp flax seed oil

2½ cups filtered water

1. In a food processor or blender, use the "high" setting and pureé all ingredients until smooth.

2. Pour into glasses and serve.

Makes: 4 (1½ cup servings)
Preparation time: 10 minutes or less
Serving size: 1½ cups or more

Corn-Free | ~~Nut and Seed-Free~~ | **Nut or Seed-Free** | **Soy-Free**

AMOUNT PER 1½ CUP SERVING: Calories 350; Calories from Fat 190; Total Fat 21g; Saturated Fat 2g; Trans Fat 0g; Cholesterol 0mg; Sodium 150mg; Total Carbohydrate 27g; Dietary Fiber 6g; Sugars 12g; Protein 16g; Vitamin A 45% DV; Vitamin C 35% DV; Calcium 15% DV; Iron 25% DV. *Recipe analyzed with 2 cups raw almond milk without dates.*

APPLE BLUE SMOOTHIE (RAW)

Protein, iron, zinc and greens are featured in this nutrient-dense flavorful drink. Bananas contain both B vitamins and potassium.

2 cups filtered water

½ head organic Romaine lettuce

½ organic apple

¼ cup frozen organic blueberries

2 frozen bananas

1 Tbsp raw black or plain sesame seeds

2 Tbsp raw pumpkin seeds

¼ cup (1 scoop) Sun Warrior Chocolate Protein®

½ Tbsp maca powder

½ Tbsp lucuma powder

1. In a food processor or blender, use the "high" setting and pureé all ingredients until smooth.

2. Pour into glasses and serve.

Makes: 4 (1½ cup servings)
Preparation time: 10 minutes or less
Serving size: 1½ cups or more

Corn-Free | ~~*Nut and Seed-Free*~~ | *Nut or Seed-Free* | *Soy-Free*

AMOUNT PER 1½ CUP SERVING: Calories 140; Calories from Fat 40;
Total Fat 4.5g; Saturated Fat .5g; Trans Fat 0g; Cholesterol 0mg; Sodium
20mg; Total Carbohydrate 22g; Dietary Fiber 3g; Sugars 11g; Protein 7g;
Vitamin A 6% DV ; Vitamin C 10% DV; Calcium 2% DV; Iron 10% DV.
Recipe analyzed with plain sesame seeds and Sun Warrior Protein®.

BANANA BLUEBERRY SMOOTHIE (RAW)

Bananas and blueberries always go well together. Strawberries add extra sweetness and vitamin C. This smoothie is easy to digest and has much more flavor than a salad made from seven leaves of lettuce.

This recipe is pictured on the cover.

1 banana

2 cups filtered water

½ cup frozen organic strawberries

½ cup frozen organic blueberries

7 organic Romaine lettuce leaves

¼ cup (1 scoop) Sun Warrior Vanilla Protein[R] or ¼ cup (2 scoops)
Raw Power!™ Protein Superfood Supplement

½ Tbsp maca powder

½ Tbsp lucuma powder

1 Tbsp hempseeds

1 Tbsp flax seed oil or hemp oil

Liquid stevia to taste

1. In a food processor or blender, use the "high" setting and pureé all ingredients until smooth.

2. Pour into glasses and serve.

Makes: 4 (1½ cup servings)
Preparation time: 10 minutes or less
Serving size: 1½ cups or more

Corn-Free | *Nut and Seed-Free* | *Nut or Seed-Free* | *Soy-Free*

HINTS, TIPS AND SUBSTITUTIONS

Raw Power!™ Protein Superfood Supplement also works well in this recipe.

Raw Power!™ Protein Superfood Supplement contains nut protein. Do not use if you are sensitive to nuts.

Omit hempseeds if you are sensitive to seeds.

AMOUNT PER 1 ½ CUP SERVING: Calories 130; Calories from Fat 50; Total Fat 5g; Saturated Fat 0g; Trans Fat 0g; Cholesterol 0mg; Sodium 15mg; Total Carbohydrate 17g; Dietary Fiber 3g; Sugars 9g; Protein 4g; Vitamin A 6% DV; Vitamin C 20% DV; Calcium 4% DV; Iron 10% DV. *Recipe analyzed with Raw Power! ™ Protein and flax oil.*

DIVE INTO YOUR DAY SMOOTHIE (RAW)

A blend of bittersweet and a hint of ginger. This provides magic for our taste buds, appealing to all of our senses. Chromium, calcium, vitamin K, magnesium and other nutrients are featured in this delicious and unusual smoothie.

2 cups filtered water

½ head of endive

¼ cup (1 scoop) Sun Warrior Chocolate Protein[R]

⅛ cup (about 2-3 Tbsp) raw organic pumpkin seeds

1½ cups organic green grapes, stems removed

1 tsp fresh ginger, minced (*If you have a high speed blender, you can use ¼ - ½-inch piece to be minced with the blending.*)

1/16 cup (½ scoop) Raw Power!™ Vanilla Protein Superfood Supplement

½ frozen banana

½ cup raw nut or seed milk (*See page 256 for recipe basics.*)

1 Tbsp acai powder

¼ tsp spirulina powder

1. In a food processor or blender, use the "high" setting and pureé all ingredients until smooth.

2. Pour into glasses and serve.

Makes: 4 (1½ cup servings)
Preparation time: 10 minutes or less
Serving size: 1½ cups or more

Corn-Free | ~~Nut and Seed-Free~~ | **Nut or Seed-Free** | **Soy-Free**

HINTS, TIPS AND SUBSTITUTIONS

If you are sensitive to seeds, use raw nut milk and omit pumpkin seeds.

Raw Power!™ Protein Superfood Supplement contains nut protein. Do not use if you are sensitive to nuts. Substitute with a different protein powder.

AMOUNT PER 1½ CUP SERVING. Calories 190; Calories from Fat 90; Total Fat 9g; Saturated Fat 2g; Trans Fat 0g; Cholesterol 0mg; Sodium 25mg; Total Carbohydrate 19g; Dietary Fiber 4g; Sugars 12g; Protein 9g; Vitamin C 15% DV; Calcium 6% DV; Iron 15% DV. *Recipe analyzed with 3 Tbsp pumpkin seeds and ½ cup raw almond milk without dates.*

GA GA GOJI COCONUT SMOOTHIE (RAW)

We often say in our home "gojis make you go go go" and this smoothie will! Though this treat contains just a few ingredients, it's packed with nutrients. May be enjoyed with hemp protein or a sweeter protein powder

1 organic kale leaf

Large handful goji berries (about ¼ cup)

2 organic celery stalks

4 Tbsp hemp protein powder

1 Tbsp flax seed oil

1 cup raw coconut water (or add another cup of filtered water)

1 cup filtered water

2 frozen bananas

1. In a food processor or blender, use the "high" setting and pureé all ingredients until smooth.

2. Pour into glasses and serve.

Makes: 4 (1½ cup servings)
Preparation time: 10 minutes or less
Serving size: 1½ cups or more

Corn-Free | Nut and Seed-Free | Nut or Seed-Free | Soy-Free

HINTS, TIPS AND SUBSTITUTIONS

Hemp protein powder gives this smoothie a "greener taste." If you prefer a sweeter taste or are sensitive to seeds, substitute Sun Warrior Protein[R] or the Raw Power!™ Protein Superfood Supplement.

Raw Power!™ Protein Superfood Supplement contains nut protein. Do not use if you are sensitive to nuts.

After blending the smoothie, add stevia if desired.

AMOUNT PER 1½ CUP SERVING: Calories 160; Calories from Fat 40; Total Fat 4.5g; Saturated Fat 0g; Trans Fat 0g; Cholesterol 0mg; Sodium 125mg; Total Carbohydrate 25g; Dietary Fiber 6g; Sugars 14g; Protein 6g; Vitamin A 15%; Vitamin C 25% DV; Calcium 4% DV; Iron 10% DV. *Recipe analyzed with 1 cup coconut water.*

PEACHY KEEN SMOOTHIE (RAW)

The peaches and bok choy will provide you with extra vitamin C, vitamin A and calcium. Using a variety of fruits and vegetables in your daily smoothies can offer you ways to obtain important nutrients throughout the week.

The Peachy Keen Smoothie pictured on the cover was made without spirulina powder.

2 - 3 cups filtered water

2 bananas *(Frozen bananas give the smoothie a thicker texture and a colder temperature.)*

1 handful (about ¼ cup) organic raw sunflower seeds

¼ tsp spirulina powder

1 leaf bok choy

¼ tsp lucuma powder

¼ tsp mesquite powder

¼ cup (1 scoop) Sun Warrior Natural Protein®

1 cup frozen organic peaches

1 Tbsp flax seed oil

1. In a food processor or blender, use the "high" setting and pureé all ingredients until smooth.

2. Pour into glasses and serve.

Makes: 4 (1½ cup servings)
Preparation time: 10 minutes or less
Serving size: 1½ cups or more

Corn-Free | *Nut and Seed-Free* | *Nut or Seed-Free* | *Soy-Free*

HINTS, TIPS AND SUBSTITUTIONS

Omit sunflower seeds if you are sensitive to seeds.

AMOUNT PER 1½ CUP SERVING: Calories 160; Calories from Fat 70; Total Fat 8g; Saturated Fat 0.5g; Trans Fat 0g; Cholesterol 0mg; Sodium 40mg; Total Carbohydrate 20g; Dietary Fiber 3g; Sugars 11g; Protein 7g; Vitamin A 6%; Vitamin C 70% DV; Calcium 4% DV; Iron 10% DV. *Recipe analyzed with 2 cups filtered water.*

RAVING RADISHES SMOOTHIE (RAW)

"Try it, you'll like it" comes to mind here. You may be pleasantly surprised. The ingredients blend well together resulting in a tasty smoothie. This happens to be one of my favorites.

4 radishes

3 beet green leaves

1 cup organic strawberries (can be frozen)

2 frozen bananas

¼ cup (1 scoop) Sun Warrior Chocolate Protein®

1 tsp lucuma powder

1 tsp maca powder

¼ tsp spirulina powder

2 -3 cups filtered water

1 Tbsp flax seed oil or hemp oil

1. In a food processor or blender, use the "high" setting and pureé all ingredients until smooth.

2. Pour into glasses and serve.

Makes: 4 (1½ cup servings)
Preparation time: 10 minutes or less
Serving size: 1½ cups or more

Corn-Free | Nut and Seed-Free | Nut or Seed-Free | Soy-Free

HINTS, TIPS AND SUBSTITUTIONS

You can substitute Raw Power!™ Chocolate Protein Superfood Supplement, and add stevia to suit your taste.

Raw Power!™ Protein Superfood Supplement contains nut protein. Do not use if you are sensitive to nuts.

AMOUNT PER 1½ CUP SERVING: Calories 130; Calories from Fat 35; Total Fat 4g; Saturated Fat 0g; Trans Fat 0g; Cholesterol 0mg; Sodium 75mg; Total Carbohydrate 20g; Dietary Fiber 4g; Sugars 10g; Protein 5g; Vitamin A 30%; Vitamin C 60% DV; Calcium 6% DV; Iron 10% DV. *Recipe analyzed with flax seed oil.*

TROPICAL GREEN SMOOTHIE (RAW)

Here you can eat your peas in smoothie form-providing B vitamins, potassium and calcium. Pineapple contains bromelain, a natural anti-inflammatory enzyme, and manganese, an important trace mineral.

¾ cup frozen pineapple

1½ frozen bananas

Large handful goji berries (about ¼ cup or up to ½ cup)

3 Tbsp dehydrated coconut "meat" from a Thai young coconut, shredded
    or finely ground

1 cup frozen peas

3 cubes frozen wheatgrass (0.6 oz. each)

2 cups raw nut or seed milk (*See page 256 for recipe basics.*)

½ cup (2 scoops) plus 2 Tbsp Sun Warrior Vanilla Protein®

1 ¼ cups filtered water or to suit desired texture/consistency

1. In a food processor or blender, use the "high" setting and pureé all ingredients until smooth.

2. Pour into glasses and serve.

Makes: 4 (1½ cup servings)
Preparation time: 10 minutes or less
Serving size: 1½ cups or more

Corn-Free | ~~*Nut and Seed-Free*~~ | *Nut or Seed-Free* | *Soy-Free*

HINTS, TIPS AND SUBSTITUTIONS

You can substitute a raw soaked grain milk if you are sensitive to nuts and seeds.

AMOUNT PER 1½ CUP SERVING: Calories 350; Calories from Fat 150; Total Fat 17g; Saturated Fat 4.5g; Trans Fat 0g; Cholesterol 0mg; Sodium 160mg; Total Carbohydrate 38g; Dietary Fiber 8g; Sugars 21g; Protein 21g; Vitamin A 2%; Vitamin C 35% DV; Calcium 10% DV; Iron 25% DV. *Recipe analyzed with ½ cup goji berries, 2 cups raw almond milk (recipe noted on page 256, excluding dates) and 1¼ cup filtered water.*

BANANA AVOCADO PUDDING (RAW)

Soothing, light, and simple to make. A nice snack or breakfast side dish.

This recipe is pictured on the cover (as a smoothie).

¼ cup mashed avocado

2 medium frozen bananas

¼ cup raw coconut *cream* (not oil)

1. Use a food processor or blender and blend together the banana and avocado.

2. Once the banana and avocado are blended, add coconut cream and blend to a creamy consistency.

3. Serve right away.

Makes: Approx. 1½ cups
Preparation time: 10 minutes
Serving size: ½ cup

Corn-Free | *Nut and Seed-Free* | *Nut or Seed-Free* | *Soy-Free*

AMOUNT PER ½ CUP SERVING: Calories 160; Calories from Fat 80; Total Fat 9g; Saturated Fat 7g; Trans Fat 0g; Cholesterol 0mg; Sodium 0mg; Total Carbohydrate 20g; Dietary Fiber 3g; Sugars 10g; Protein 2g; Vitamin A 2% DV; Vitamin C 15% DV; Iron 4% DV.

CREAMY FRUIT PUDDING (RAW)

*This dessert blends fruit and fat without elevating blood sugar.
Choose your favorite fruits and make an array of delectable creations.*

¾ cup favorite fruit (*Peel and core organic apples, organic pears, organic peaches and oranges before blending.*)

2 Tbsp raw coconut *cream* (not oil)

Filtered water, raw coconut water or raw nut milk to desired consistency

Add liquid stevia to taste

1. Combine all ingredients in a blender and blend until thoroughly mixed.

2. For best results, serve right away. Store additional pudding in the refrigerator. Will keep for 2-3 days in an airtight container.

Makes: Approx. 1½ cups
Preparation time: 10 minutes or less
Serving size: ½ cup

Corn-Free | *Nut and Seed-Free* | *Nut or Seed-Free* | *Soy-Free*

AMOUNT PER ½ CUP SERVING: Calories 80; Calories from Fat 35; Total Fat 3.5g; Saturated Fat 3g; Trans Fat 0g; Cholesterol 0mg; Sodium 0mg; Total Carbohydrate 14g; Dietary Fiber 2g; Sugars 7g; Protein 1g; Vitamin C 8% DV; Iron 2% DV. *Recipe analyzed with ¾ cup banana and coconut cream only.*

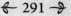

PART 3

Appendix

and Resources

*These products can be useful when making recipes for vegans or those with food
sensitivities. I do not work for any of these companies, but occasionally, when I
believe in a product, I become an affiliate. I hope these suggestions help you. I
encourage you to ask your local retailers to special order and/or carry these
products for you. Although some brands listed may also manufacture other
well-made products, I am endorsing only the products noted here.*

If you have trouble finding any of the listed
items, please feel free to contact me
for the most current source listing.

Alternative Sweetener Sources

❀ **AGAVE NECTAR SYRUP** is available through a number of sources. The Wholesome Sweetener® Company's blue agave has been processed with low temperature evaporation and uses fair trade practices. Madhava™ Honey uses an organic enzyme at a low temperature to process their agave nectar. Both Volcanic Nectar™ Blue Agave (which is free of corn syrup) and Sweet Cactus Farms® claim to be safe for diabetics. All of these companies claim their nectars are organic. Many raw food enthusiasts use clear agave nectar. Please see my recommendation for agave nectar use in Chapter 12 beginning on page 73. *www.wholesomesweeteners.com, www.madhavahoney.com, www.globalgoods.com* and *www.sweetcactusfarms.com.*

❀ **BARLEY MALT** is available through Eden® Organic and Great Eastern Sun Sweet Cloud® brand. *www.edenfoods.com* and *www.great-eastern-sun.com.*

❀ **BROWN RICE SYRUP** is available through Eden Organic®, Great Eastern Sun Sweet Cloud®, and Lundberg Family Farms Organic Sweet Dreams®. *www.edenfoods.com, www.great-eastern-sun.com* and *www.lundberg.com.*

❀ **COCONUT SUGAR** is available through Coconut Secret®, Navitas Naturals®, SweetTree Sustainable Sweeteners™, and Wilderness Family Naturals®. *www.coconutsecret.com, www.navitasnaturals.com, www.sweet-tree.biz* and *www.wildernessfamilynaturals.com.*

❀ **DATE SUGAR** functions as both sweetener and binder. It is most effective to soak organic pitted dates for twenty to thirty minutes, and grind them yourself before adding them to recipes. Date sugar is available in a granulated form through Bob's Red Mill® and Chatfield's®. *www.chatfieldsbrand.com* and *www.bobsredmill.com.*

❋ **Frozen Fruit Concentrates and Fruit Spreads** are available in organic and non-organic varieties. Please note some of these brands are owned by large corporations. See pages 117-118 for more information.

Non-organic varieties include:
Dickinson's Purely Fruit® *(www.dickinsonsfamily.com)*
Polaner All Fruit Spreads® *(www.polanerallfruit.com)*
Smucker's Simply 100% Fruit® *(www.smuckers.com)*
St. Dalfour Fruit Conserves® *(www.stdalfour.us)*
Tree of Life Fruit Spread® *(www.treeoflife.com)*

Organic varieties include:
Bionaturae® *(www.bionaturae.com)*
Crofter's® Organic fruit spread *(www.croftersorganic.com)*
R.W. Knudsen Family® *(www.rwknudsenfamily.com)*

Please check food labels because many of these companies make spreads using corn syrup, sugar, and Splenda®. Some also contain fruit syrups and/ or ascorbic acid (which may be corn-derived).

❋ **Honey** is best purchased from your local beekeepers who can teach you about their beekeeping processes. Other brands include: Really Raw®, Ambrosia® Honey Products (by Madhava™), and The Synergy Company™ Manuka Healing Honey. *www.reallyrawhoney.com, www.madhavahoney.com* and *www.thesynergycompany.com.*

❋ **Jerusalem Artichoke Syrup** is currently difficult to find. I am looking for a reputable source. Contact me for more information.

❋ **Maple Sugar Crystals** are available through Shady Maple Farms®. *www.shadymaple.ca.*

❋ **Maple syrup** is available unprocessed (without added corn syrup or sweetener) through a variety of sources. Look for local organic sources closest to where you live. Other ideas include: Shady Maple Farms®, Maple Valley Maple Products®, Strawberry

Hill Farms®. *www.shadymaple.ca, www.maplevalleysyrup.com* and *www.puremaple.com.*

❋ **Molasses** is available through The Wholesome Sweetener® Company. *www.wholesomesweeteners.com.*

❋ **Rapadura**® is available through Rapunzel®. *www.rapunzel.com.*

❋ **Stevia** brands listed below are currently produced without the use of harmful chemicals and additional ingredients (e.g. maltodextrin, erythritol, etc.) Filtered water is used during production.

> **Body Ecology Diet**® **Stevia Liquid Concentrate**: *www.bodyecologydiet.com.*

> **NuNaturals, Inc.** offers NuStevia™ White Stevia™ Extract Powder, Pure Liquid™ Alcohol-Free Stevia™ (glass bottle), Pure Liquid™ Clear Stevia™ (glass bottle), Pure Liquid™ Vanilla Alcohol-Free Stevia™ and NuStevia™ White Stevia™ Quick Dissolve Tabs. *www.nunaturals.com.*

> **SweetLeaf**™ prepares flavored SteviaClear® liquid stevia, available in Vanilla Crème, Chocolate Raspberry, Lemon Drop, Valencia Orange, Cinnamon, Grape, Chocolate, Peppermint, Root Beer, Apricot Nectar, and English Toffee. *www.sweetleaf.com.*

> **SweetLeaf**™ also offers SteviaPlus® and Stevia Concentrate Dark Liquid®. *www.sweetleaf.com.*

> **Young Living Essentials**® *www.youngliving.com.*

❋ **Tapioca syrup** is available through Nature's Flavors' and Barry Farm Foods. *www.naturesflavors.com* and *www.barryfarm.com.*

❋ **Xylitol** derived from birch only is recommended. A few brands include Designs for Health®, Smart Sweet® and The Ultimate Sweetener®. Contact me for more information.

❋ **Yacon syrup** is available through a variety of companies such as Natural Zing®, Navitas Naturals® and Raw Food World®. At the time of this writing, most companies processing yacon are making it without the use of additives and preservatives. Please see the websites listed on page 314.

Gluten-Free Baking Mixes, Flours and Oats

Some gluten-free flours containing high amounts of rice, potato, arrowroot, cornstarch and other higher-glycemic grains may raise blood sugar more than bean-based gluten-free flours. If you are a diabetic, please check your blood sugar upon consumption and experiment to find what works for you.

❋ **Arrowhead Mills**® carries an array of gluten-free flours, including All Purpose Baking Mix and Pancake and Waffle Mix. This company is owned by The Hain Celestial Group®. A percentage of their products are also owned by Heinz®. See pages 117-118 for more information. *www.arrowheadmills.com.*

❋ **Bob's Red Mill**® carries a wide variety of allergen-free products including cereals and flours (e.g. brown rice, almond, hazelnut, teff and millet). The Gluten-Free All Purpose Baking Flour Mix does not contain corn, baking powder or baking soda and it has a slightly "beany" flavor. *www.bobsredmill.com.*

❋ **Gifts of Nature**™ offers an All Purpose Flour Blend and Certified Gluten-Free Rolled Oats and Whole Groats. The flour blend does not contain corn, baking powder or baking soda, and it has a slightly "beany" flavor. *www.giftsofnature.net.*

❋ **Gluten Evolution Breads from Anna**® carries a wide variety of bread and muffin mixes sweetened with honey or maple sugar. Most products are free of many common allergens. Check ingredients before using. Eggs may be needed for preparation. *www.breadsfromanna.com.*

❋ **Gluten Free Essentials**® carries an All Purpose Baking Mix containing organic rice flour and non-GMO sorghum flour. Some products contain cornstarch, soy, or dairy products. *www.gfessentials.com.*

❈ **Namaste Foods**[R]**, LLC** carries a Perfect Flour Blend, a Biscuits, Piecrust and More Blend, Waffle and Pancake Mix, and a Sugar-Free Muffin Mix. *www.namastefoods.com.*

❈ **Shiloh Farms**[R] carries different whole grain flours, many of which are allergen-free. *www.shilohfarms.com.*

Gluten-Free Oats

❈ **Bob's Red Mill**[R] carries certified organic rolled oats and a variety of other products. *www.bobsredmill.com.*

❈ **Cream Hill Estates (Lara's Gluten-Free)**[R] carries certified organic oat groats, rolled oats and oat flour. *www.creamhillestates.com.*

❈ **Gifts of Nature**[R] carries certified gluten-free oats and oat products. *www.giftsofnature.net.*

Baking Products

❈ **Alcohol-free extracts and/or flavorings** are available in a variety of flavors through the Frontier[TM] and Simply Organic[R] brands. *If you are sensitive to corn, check with the manufacturer to be sure corn alcohol is not used. Frontier[TM] extracts may contain corn alcohol. www.frontiercoop.com* and *www.simplyorganicfoods.com.*

❈ **Allergy-free, dairy-free chocolate or carob chips** are available through Enjoy Life Foods[R] (contains cane juice); Sunspire[R] (their grain-sweetened chocolate chips contain barley, corn and soy lecithin; their carob chips contain barley, corn and soy lecithin); and Tropical Source[R] chips (contain cane juice and soy lecithin). *www.enjoylifefoods.com, www.sunspire.com* and *www.worldpantry.com.*

❈ **Aluminum-free baking powder** is available through Rumford[R], Featherweight[R], or Bob's Red Mill[R]. Featherweight[R] makes a corn-free baking powder. *www.clabbergirl.com, www.hainpurefoods.com* and *www.bobsredmill.com.*

❋ **CELTIC SEA SALT**[R] is available through The Grain & Salt Society[R] and Flower of the Ocean[R]. This salt has many viable nutrients not contained in standard table salt. *www.celticseasalt.com.*

❋ **CHEWING GUMS** that contain xylitol from birch are XyliChew[R] and Xponent[R] gums. These products contain beeswax. Companies that manufacture these products may also make products containing non-recommended sweeteners. B Fresh Gum is a vegan gum, also containing xylitol made from birch. *www.tundratrading. com, www.globalsweet.com* and *www.bfreshgum.com.*

❋ **COCONUT CREAM** is available through Artisana[R], Cocopura[R], Let's Do…Organic[R], or Tropical Traditions[R]. Also see websites listed on page 314. *www.edwardandsons.com.*

❋ **COCONUT MILK** is available through Native Forest[R] and Thai Kitchen[R]. *www.edwardandsons.com* and *www.thaikitchen.com.*

❋ **COCONUT OIL** is available through Artisana[R], Cocopura[R], LoveRawFoods[TM], Nutiva[R], Tropical Traditions[R] or Tropics Best[R]. See websites listed on page 314.

❋ **COCONUT WATER** is available through Edward & Sons[R] and O.N.E.[TM] *www.edwardandsons.com* and *www.onenaturalexperience.com.*

❋ **DAIRY-FREE, GLUTEN-FREE, SOY-FREE ICE CREAMS:** Remember to check food labels because manufacturers change ingredients and formulas without notice. Some of these products may contain xanthan gum and/or soy lecithin. Sweetened varieties may contain cane sugar.

> **Blue Mountain Organics**[R] makes Raw and Organic Cashew Creamery[TM] in a variety of flavors. They are agave and lucuma-sweetened and are soy-free. *www.bluemountainorganics.com.*

> **Luna & Larry's Coconut Bliss**[R] is organic and available in a variety of flavors. These are sweetened with agave nectar. *www.coconutbliss.com.*

(continued)

❋ **Dairy-free, gluten-free, soy-free ice creams:** (continued)

Purely Decadent[R] comes in a variety of flavors from Turtle Mountain[R]. These frozen treats are made with coconut milk and sweetened with agave. This brand also makes a fudge bar and ice pop. Turtle Mountain also manufactures a line containing soy. *www.sodeliciousdairyfree.com.*

❋ **Dairy-free, gluten-free milks:** Remember to check food labels because manufacturers change ingredients and formulas without notice. Some of these products may contain xanthan gum and/or soy lecithin. Sweetened varieties may contain cane sugar. Some of these brands are owned by large corporations. See pages 117-118 for more information.

Almond milk is available through Blue Diamond Growers[R] Almond Breeze, Pacific Natural Foods[R] and The Hain Celestial Group[R], Inc. (Almond Dream™). *www.bluediamondgrowers.com, www.pacificfoods.com and www.hain-celestial.com.*

Hemp milk is available through Living Harvest[R] (Tempt™ Hemp Milk), Manitoba Harvest[R] (Hemp Bliss™), Pacific Natural Foods[R] and the The Hain Celestial Group[R], Inc. (Hemp Dream™). *www.livingharvest.com, www.manitobaharvest.com, www.pacificfoods.com and www.hain-celestial.com.*

Rice milk is available through Good Karma[R] (Whole Grain Organic Rice Milk), Pacific Natural Foods[R] and The Hain Celestial Group[R], Inc. (Rice Dream™) If you are on a strict gluten-free diet, Rice Dream™ may be rinsed/washed with barley. *www.goodkarmafoods.com, www.pacificfoods.com and www.hain-celestial.com.*

❋ **Dairy-free, gluten-free yogurts:** Some of these brands are owned by large corporations. See pages 117-118 for more information.

Nancy's[R] **Organic** cultured soy yogurt is vegan, wheat-free and contains soy. It is sweetened with amasake, white grape juice, pure maple syrup or agave to sweeten. *Nancy's*[R] *also sells cultured dairy products.* www.nancysyogurt.com.

Ricera[R] is a vegan rice-based yogurt that is soy-free, dairy-free and wheat-free and contains cane sugar. Recommended only for occasional consumption. *www.ricerafoods.com.*

Turtle Mountain So Delicious[R] **Coconut Milk Yogurt** is vegan, soy-free and dairy-free, and contains both dextrose and cane sugar. Recommended only for occasional consumption. *This company makes soy products and other coconut products.* www.soydelicious.com.

WholeSoy & Co.[R] yogurt contains organic soy, organic cane juice and organic cornstarch. Recommended only for occasional consumption. *www.wholesoyco.com.*

WildWood Organics[TM] organic soy yogurt makes a plain unsweetened flavor containing dextrose (for the probiotic culture). Some flavors are sweetened with organic cane juice and dextrose and are only recommended for occasional consumption. *www.pulmuonewildwood.com.*

❋ **Dried organic fruit** is available through Eden Organic[R], GoHunza[R] and LoveRawFoods[TM]. Some of these fruits are sweetened. *www.edenfoods.com, www.GoHunza.com* and *www.bluemountainorganics.com.*

❋ **Excalibur**[R] **dehydrators** are versatile machines that offer flexibility in the kitchen. They can be used to dry herbs, nuts and seeds; and make raw sweet treats, crackers, homemade dried fruit and fruit "leather". To learn more or place an order, visit *www.SweetnessWithoutSugar.com*.

❋ **Fresh fruits and vegetables** can be found at your local farmer's market. See page 120 if you are interested in learning about the fruits and vegetables with the highest and lowest amounts of pesticides. Search *www.localharvest.org* to find a farmer's market near you.

❋ **Himalayan salt** is available through The Original Himalayan Crystal Salt[R] and HimalaSalt[TM]. *www.himalayancrystalsalt.com* and *www.himalasalt.com*.

❋ **Multi-Pure**[R] **Drinking Water Systems** offer reverse osmosis stainless steel models for your sinktop or below-the-sink installation. This company provides a solid and certified (by The National Safety Foundation) alternative to bottled waters and contaminated city drinking water. Using a filter produces less waste and toxic load than that generated by using unrecyclable plastic bottles. If we drink liquids stored in unrecyclable plastic bottles, we can ingest undesirable pollutants. To learn more or place an order, visit *www.SweetnessWithoutSugar.com*.

❋ **Natural Decorating Colors** are available through India Tree[R] and The Original Family Herb Tea Company[R]. They make colors created with vegetable colorants, a non-toxic option for coloring your sweet treats! Let's Do...Organic[R] makes gluten-free and natural Sprinkelz[TM] to top your treats. *www.indiatree.com, www.seelectea.com* and *www.edwardandsons.com*

❋ **Nut and Seed Butters** are available through a variety
of resources. Most of the raw versions are unsweetened and
unsalted. Some of these choices are organic. Some of these
brands are owned by large corporations. See pages 117-118 for
more information.

Raw choices include:
Artisana^R *(www.premierorganics.org)*
Better Than Roasted™
    (www.bluemountainorganics.com/betterthanroasted/)
Futters Nut Butters™ *(www.futtersnutbutters.com)*
LoveRawFoods™ *(www.bluemountainorganics.com)*
Marantha^R *(www.maranathafoods.com)*
Rejuvenative Foods^R *(www.rejuvenative.com)*
Trader Joe's^R *(www.traderjoes.com)*
Tree of Life^R *(treeoflife.com)*
Wilderness Poets^R *(www.wildernesspoets.com)*

Roasted choices include:
Futters Nut Butters™ *(www.futtersnutbutters.com)*
Marantha^R *(www.maranathafoods.com)*
SunButter^R *(www.sunbutter.com)*
365 Whole Foods^R brand *(www.wholefoodsmarket.com)*

❋ **Organic flax seeds** (golden or brown) are available whole
or pre-ground through Bob's Red Mill^R. Sprouted flax seeds
are available plain and with fruits through Sprout Revolution™.
www.bobsredmill.com and *www.puravidaproducts.com*.

❋ **Protein Powders**
Hemp protein powders containing organic hemp protein:
Living Harvest^R *(www.livingharvest.com)*
Nutiva^R *(www.nutiva.com)*
Ruth's Hemp Foods^R *(www.ruthshempfoods.com)*
Manitoba Harvest^R *(www.manitobaharvest.com)*
North Coast Naturals^R *(www.northcoastnaturals.com)*

❋ **Protein Powders** (continued):

Mixed blend protein powders:

Peaceful Planet Inca Meal™ by VegLife® is a raw sprouted rice protein blend. It also contains amaranth, quinoa, maca, chia and a variety of fruits. This blend is organic and sweetened with yacon and stevia. *www.veganessentials.com.*

Peaceful Planet The Supreme Meal™ by VegLife® is a blend of high-protein grains, rice and pea protein, and superfoods. Offer this to children 3+ years old *only* after ensuring that they tolerate grains, rice, peas and superfoods. This product contains lecithin (which is derived from soy). *www.veganessentials.com.*

Potent Proteins by Body Ecology™ contains a variety of organic, fermented superfoods including spirulina, brown rice, millet, quinoa, chickpeas, soybeans, flax seeds and alfalfa seeds. *www.bodyecologydiet.com.*

Raw Power!™ **Protein Superfood Supplement!**® contains a raw protein blend including hempseed, maca, Brazil nut and more. Available in chocolate, vanilla, natural and green. Because this product has a pleasant texture and flavor, I recommend it to people who wish to add more raw foods into their diets. *www.rawpower.com.*

Sproutein™ is a raw protein blend of sprouts, superfoods, fruits and vegetables. It contains omega oils from hemp and chia and is sweetened with lucuma and yacon. *www.sproutliving.com*

Vega® **Whole Food Health Optimizer** is a mixture of brown rice, hemp and yellow pea proteins. This product comes in different flavors. Vanilla Chai is a personal favorite. To determine your favorite flavors, try packet-sizes first. Incorporate this into a child's (3+ years old) diet *only* after making sure the child has no sensitivities to individual ingredients in this product. *www.sequelnaturals.com.*

RAW PROTEIN POWDERS:

Peaceful Planet Inca Meal™ by VegLife® is a raw sprouted rice protein blend. It also contains amaranth, quinoa, maca, chia and a variety of fruits. This blend is organic and sweetened with yacon and stevia. *www.veganessentials.com.*

Raw Power!™ **Protein Superfood Supplement!**® contains a raw protein blend including hempseed, maca, Brazil nut and more. Available in chocolate, vanilla, natural and green. Because this product has a pleasant texture and flavor, I recommend it to people who wish to add more raw foods into their diets. *www.rawpower.com.*

Sproutein™ is a raw protein blend of sprouts, superfoods, fruits and vegetables. It contains omega oils from hemp and chia and is sweetened with lucuma and yacon. *www.sproutliving.com.*

Sun Warrior Protein® is a raw protein powder which is made from brown rice and contains stevia as a sweetener. Three flavors are available: natural, vanilla and chocolate. All flavors are tasty and have a nice texture. *www.sunwarrior.com.*

RICE PROTEIN POWDERS: *Some of these brands are owned by large corporations. See pages 117-118 for more information.*

Nutribiotic® **Rice Protein** is made from brown rice and is available in chocolate, vanilla, natural, mixed berry, with flaxseed, and with antioxidants. This company (Biochem®) also makes a vegan protein with a combination of hemp, yellow pea and cranberry protein called 100% Vegan Protein. *www.nutribiotic.com.*

(continued)

❋ **PROTEIN POWDERS:** (continued)

RICE PROTEIN POWDERS (continued):

Organic Brown Rice Protein by North Coast Naturals[R] is made from GMO-free, certified organic brown rice. *www.veganessentials.com.*

Sun Warrior Protein[R] is a raw protein powder which is made from brown rice and contains stevia as a sweetener. Three flavors are available: natural, vanilla and chocolate. All flavors are tasty and have a nice texture. *www.sunwarrior.com.*

❋ **QUINOA FLAKES** are available through Ancient Harvest[R], a company that carries a wide variety of quinoa products. *www.quinoa.net.*

❋ **STAINLESS STEEL BAKING PRODUCTS** are available through Organic Grace[R]. The quality of stainless steel is an important factor when purchasing stainless steel products. Life Without Plastic[TM] and Happy Tiffin[TM] also offer stainless products for tableware, lunchboxes and more. *www.organicgrace.com, www.lifewithoutplastic.com* and *www.happytiffin.com.*

❋ **UNSWEETENED JUICE** is available through Lakewood[R] Juices and Woodstock Farms[R]. They offer a wide range of organic, unsweetened juices and concentrates free from ascorbic acid. *www.lakewoodjuices.com* and *www.woodstock-farms.com.*

❋ **UNSWEETENED, ALKALI-FREE AND DAIRY-FREE COCOAS** are found in the following brands including: Ahlaska[R], Chatfield's[R], and Rapunzel[R]. *www.ahlaska.com, www.chatfieldsbrand.com* and *www.rapunzel.com.* Dairy-free carob is available through *Chatfield's*[R].

❋ **VITAMIX**[R] is a high-speed blender that is helpful for making a variety of sweet treats, green smoothies, and other blended delicacies. *Though expensive, my Vitamix has been used frequently for seven years and has not yet required replacement.* To learn more or place an order, visit: *https://secure.vitamix.com/acb/stores/4/?COUPON=06-003827, www.vitamix.com.*

Additional Gluten-Free Sources

Breads

❈ **Chébé**[R] carries a variety of breads and doughs free from wheat, gluten, yeast, corn, peanuts, tree nuts, soy, rice and potato. Five of their bread mixes are dairy-free but require eggs for preparation. The Chebe website reports customers having success using Chebe bread mixes with egg substitutes. *www.chebe.com.*

❈ **Grindstone Bakery** carries a variety of gluten-free breads. Minimum orders are required. *www.grindstonebakery.com.*

❈ **Sami's Bakery**[R] carries a wide variety of gluten-free breads, crackers, tortillas and more. They use mostly millet, flax and brown rice in their products. I do not recommend their sweet products which contain mostly fructose. *www.samisbakery.com.*

Websites

❈ **The following websites** offer an array of gluten-free products. Be sure to check product ingredients; some may not be sugar-free or use alternative sweeteners. However, if you are new to living with food sensitivities, you can see by examining these websites that you definitely have options! Ask your local retailers to carry these products for you.

> *www.glutenfreemall.com*
> *www.missroben.com*
> *www.glutenfreepantry.com*
> *www.celiac.com*
> *www.namastefoods.com*
> *www.glutenfree.com*
> *www.gluten.net*
> *www.cherrybrookkitchen.com*

Energy Bars Containing Alternative Sweeteners

Consider buying these products at your local health food stores. Unless otherwise noted, all bars are gluten-, dairy- and soy-free.

Many of these bars contain agave nectar and/or organic cane sugar. Please check the labels to ensure the ingredients suit your needs. I have included a few options containing honey for both honey-eating vegans and those eating honey while transitioning from other sweeteners.

Vegan Options

Some of these brands are owned by large corporations. See pages 117-118 for more information.

❋ **Cocochia**[R] bars contain TheraSweet[R] and are recommended for occasional consumption until further research is performed. *http://www.livingfuel.com/CocoChia-Snack-Fuel-Bars.aspx.*

❋ **Crenu**[R] are available in eight flavors. They are GMO-free and are sweetened with both cane sugar and agave nectar. *http://crenu.com.*

❋ **Gertrude & Bronner's Magic Alpsnack**[TM] are available in five flavors. These bars contain organic ingredients and are sweetened with organic cane sugar and rice syrup. Two varieties include Fair Trade Dark Chocolate, organic sugar and soy lecithin. *www.drbronner.com/DBMS/ALP.htm.*

❋ **Organic Cocoa Cassava Bar** is sweetened with tapioca syrup and contains chia seeds, coconut and almonds. This delicious bar has a predominantly smooth texture with a slight crunch of chia seeds. *www.products.mercola.com.*

❋ **Organic Food Bars**[R] are available in nine different varieties. Most of the bars contain agave syrup. Some contain organic cane sugar. *www.organicfoodbar.com.*

❋ **PranaBar**® is available in six flavors. Supercharger Pranabars® contain superfoods and are available in four flavors. All bars contain agave syrup. The manufacturer, Divine Foods Products™, also makes thirteen varieties of Boomi Bars™, which contain honey. *Two contain whey, which is a dairy product.* PranaBar Shakti® bars are made exclusively for Whole Foods® Market with superfoods and may contain cane sugar. *www.pranabars.com.*

❋ **Sunspire**® **Coconut Bar** is packaged in a red label and offers a dairy-free alternative to a Mounds® bar. This company has other vegan chocolate treats that contain sugar (and soy lecithin) but may be helpful for transitioning from artificial sweeteners and dairy. Some examples include the Organic Dark Chocolate Almonds, Organic Dark Chocolate Blueberries, Organic Dark Chocolate Cranberries, Organic Dark Chocolate Raisins and the Tropical Source® Toasted Almond Chocolate Bar. *The company does not guarantee these products gluten- or allergen-free.* *www.worldpantry.com.*

❋ **Vega**® by Sequel Naturals offers Whole Food Vibrancy Bars® and Whole Food Energy Bars®, both in three flavors containing agave syrup and mostly organic ingredients. All bars are GMO and pesticide-free. *Chocolate Decadence contains organic raw sugar. www.sequelnaturals.com.*

❋ **You Bar**™ is a service that lets you create your own bar and name it as you choose. Their products include nut and seed butters, protein powder, seeds, dried fruits and superfoods. Among the sweetener options are stevia and brown rice syrup. *www.youbars.com/buildabar/.*

❋ **Zing Nutrition Bars**® has created two vegan bars (e.g. Peanut Butter Chocolate Chip and Cranberry Orange) containing FruitTrim® (only available to manufacturers), agave nectar and some organic ingredients. *www.zingbars.com.*

Energy Bars Containing Alternative Sweeteners (cont.)
Raw (and Vegan) options

All of the following brands offer energy bars in a variety of flavors. Many of these bars contain agave. Please check ingredients to ensure they suit your needs.

- ❋ CCNO® BARS (www.ccnoforlife.com)

- ❋ GOPAL'S® RAWMA BARS* (www.gopalshealthfoods.com)

- ❋ JAKE'S UNBAKED BAR® or EARTHLING ORGANICS™ (www.earthlingorganics.com)

- ❋ LARABARS® Most bars contain raw ingredients. The cocoa and cashews are not guaranteed raw. One bar contains peanuts. (www.larabar.com)

- ❋ LOVE FORCE ENERGY BARS®** (www.loveforce.net)

- ❋ LYDIA'S ORGANIC® RAW BARS (www.lydiasorganics.com)

- ❋ ORGANIC FOOD® BARS are available in four raw varieties. (www.organicfoodbar.com)

- ❋ PURE® ORGANIC BARS are certified-organic. (www.thepurebar.com)

- ❋ RAW CRUNCH® BARS*** (www.kathyfeldman.com)

- ❋ RAW ORGANIC gRAWnola® BAR (www.grawnola.com)

- ❋ RAW REVOLUTION® (www.rawindulgence.com)

- ❋ RIGHTEOUSLY RAW® BARS are similar to traditional candy bars. (www.earthsourceorganics.com)

- ❋ THE RAW BAKERY™ GOJI BAR (www.bluemountainorganics.com)

- ❋ WILDBAR™ (www.wildbar.info)

---

* *Gopal's® makes another bar named Adam & Eve that contains non-gluten-free oats.*

** *Check individual ingredients. At least one flavor contains non-gluten-free oats.*

*** *Sweetened with raw honey. Do not eat if pregnant or breastfeeding. Do not feed to a child under one year of age. Not suitable for young children.*

Sweet Snacks

These are a few healthier "on the go" sweet ideas for those who travel or have busy lifestyles. You may want to ask your local retailer to carry these products. Some of these brands are owned by large corporations. See pages 117-118 for more information.

❋ **ACAI JUICE** is available (sweetened or unsweetened) in frozen "packets" in many health food stores. Eat the packet as a frozen ice pop treat or add it to a smoothie. Even with the added sugar, acai is a delicious alternative to ice pops with dairy, dyes and unhealthy fillers. *www.sambazon.com.*

❋ **AIMEE'S LIVIN' MAGIC**® makes a variety of raw, nutrient-dense, on-the-go snacks to meet many tastes. *www.aimeeslivinmagic.com.*

❋ **BETTER THAN ROASTED**™ makes a variety of Love Bites™ containing a mixture of nuts, dried fruit and spices. *www.bluemountainorganics.com.*

❋ **CACAO NIBS MIXED WITH PITTED DATES** are an easy "grab and go" snack that will satisfy your sweet tooth!

❋ **CHOCOLATE:** Examine labels to find varieties with a Fair Trade designation and at least a 70% cacao content. Vegans may seek dairy-free varieties. Chocolate may contain sugar in an alternative form. One example includes Chocolove®, which offers dark chocolate varieties made without milk. *Those with severe milk allergies should use caution when consuming these products because manufacturers may use a facility that processes milk chocolate. www.chocolove.com.*

❋ **GONE NUTS!**® makes sprouted and seasoned nuts and nut blends. *www.livingintentions.com.*

❋ **GO RAW**® snacks and cookies come in a variety of flavors. They are organic, raw and predominately gluten-free, wheat-free and nut-free. These snacks will also give you a boost of superfoods. *www.goraw.com.*

❋ **GRAINAISSANCE, INC.**® makes shakes in a variety of flavors that are easy to grab and take with you. The Mocha-Java flavor contains gluten. Some combinations contain nuts, xanthan gum, and/or non-GMO soy. *www.grainaissance.com.*

❋ **KookieKarma**® makes raw and baked snack bars and treats using whole food ingredients. Some products contain xylitol and agave nectar. *www.kookiekarma.com.*

❋ **The Raw Bakery**™ makes a variety of raw snacks, both sweet and savory. *www.bluemountainorganics.com.*

❋ **Udo's Oil**® makes a dairy-free truffle which contains essential fatty acids. *www.udoerasmus.com.*

❋ **Ulimana**® truffles sweetened with agave nectar, coconut nectar or honey are available in a variety of combinations. The company sells a small "to go" package of two. *www.ulimana.com.*

For other snack ideas, look out for *Wendy's Snack Booklet* coming soon! For details, visit www.vigdorhess.com.

Superfoods (as described on pages 67-71)

Ask your local retailers to carry these superfoods! If you prefer that I order the products for you, visit my websites, www.vigdorhess.com or www.SweetnessWithoutSugar.com. For your convenience, the websites for many of these companies are listed on page 314.

❋ **Acai** is available through Sambazon® and Navitas Naturals®.

❋ **Blue-Green Algae** is available through Tachyon®. Many other products listed here contain this superfood.

❋ **Cacao** is available through a variety of companies such as Natural Zing®, Raw Food World® and RawGuru®.

❋ **Camu camu berry** is available through a variety of companies such as Natural Zing®, Raw Food World® and RawGuru®.

❋ **Chia seeds** are available through a variety of companies such as Natural Zing®, Navitas Naturals®, Raw Food World®, RawGuru® and Ruth's Hemp®.

✳ **Coconut cream** is available through Artisana®, Cocopura® or Tropical Traditions®.

✳ **Coconut oil** is available raw through Artisana®. Tropical Traditions® and Cocopura® are other well-regulated companies that carry organic coconut oil and coconut cream. Nutiva® and Tropics Best® are other resources. With no added fillers, chemicals or flavors, coconut oil is also delicious when eaten plain.

✳ **Crystal Manna**™ is available through a variety of companies including Natural Zing® and Raw Food World® and RawGuru®.

✳ **E3 Live**™ is available through a variety of companies including Natural Zing®, Raw Food World®, and RawGuru®. It can also be ordered directly through the E3 Live™ company.

✳ **Fruits of the Earth**™ is available through Healthforce®.

✳ **Goji berries** are available through a variety of companies including Natural Zing®, Raw Food World® and RawGuru®.

✳ **Hemp seeds and protein** is available through Living Harvest®, Manitoba Harvest®, Nutiva®, and Ruth's Hemp®. *Please see page 303 for more information about hemp protein powders.* Living Harvest® and Manitoba Harvest® make organic and unsweetened hemp milk.

✳ **Lucuma powder** is available through a variety of companies including Natural Zing®, Raw Food World® and RawGuru®.

✳ **Maca root powder** is available through a variety of companies including Natural Zing®, Raw Food World® and RawGuru®.

✳ **Maqui berry** is available through RawGuru®.

✳ **Perfect Food**® **RAW Organic Green Super Food** is a product of Garden of Life®, Inc. A green vegetable juice in a powdered form.

❋ **Pure Synergy**® is a product of The Synergy Company®. It is available through a variety of companies including Natural Zing®, Raw Food World® and RawGuru®.

❋ **Spirulina powder** is available through a number of companies. I recommend the Healthforce® brand.

❋ **Vitamineral Green**™ is available through Healthforce®.

*Companies Selling Superfoods**

❋ Artisana® *(www.premierorganics.org)*

❋ Cocopura® *(www.vivapura.net)*

❋ E3Live™ *(www.e3live.com)*

❋ Healthforce® *(www.healthforce.com)*

❋ Living Harvest *(www.livingharvest.com)*

❋ Manitoba Harvest *(www.manitobaharvest.com)*

❋ Natural Zing® *(www.naturalzing.com)*

❋ Navitas Naturals® *(www.navitasnaturals.com)*

❋ Nutiva® *(www.nutiva.com)*

❋ Raw Food World® *(www.therawfoodworld.com)*

❋ Raw Guru® *(www.rawguru.com)*

❋ Raw Power® *(www.rawpower.com)*

❋ Ruth's Hemp® *(www.ruthshempfoods.com)*

❋ Sambazon® *(www.sambazon.com)*

❋ Tachyon® *(www.tachyonenergy.org)*

❋ The Synergy Company® *(www.thesynergycompany.com)*

❋ Tropical Traditions® *(www.tropicaltraditions.com)*

❋ Tropics Best® *(www.tropicsbest.com)*

---

* *If you would like to place an order, many of these links are available at www.sweetnesswithoutsugar.com*

Resources for Eating Healthfully

These documentaries, commentaries and resources reveal how our food choices impact our physical and environmental health. If you would like to know of additional titles, please contact me. I will be happy to suggest more.

* *Food Matters* (DVD): *www.foodmatters.tv/_webapp/Movie_Store.*

* *King Corn* by Michael Pollan (DVD).

* *Sweet Misery: A Poisoned World* by Cori Brackett (DVD).

* *Killer at Large: Why Obesity is America's Greatest Threat* (DVD).

* *Sweet Remedy: The World Reacts to an Adulterated Food Supply* (DVD).

* *Sugar: The Bitter Truth* by Dr. Robert Lustig, UCSF Professor of Pediatrics in the Division of Endocrinology (video): *www.youtube.com/watch?v=dBnniua6-oM.*

* *The Non-GMO Shopping Guide* is available through The Institute for Responsible Technology (IRT) and The Center for Food Safety (CFS). *www.nongmoshoppingguide.com/SG/Home/index.cfm.*

More Raw Living Sources

* *The Lazy Raw Foodist's Guide* is a wonderful guide for busy people, lazy or not. This e-book offers ideas for easy preparation of healthy foods, as well as practical tips and suggestions for maintaining good health while eating raw foods. Written by Laura Bruno, a successful Lazy Raw Foodist, Medical Intuitive, Coach and Reiki Master Teacher. *www.lazyrawfoodist.com.*

* *Simply Raw: Reversing Diabetes in 30 Days* is a documentary about people who reverse diabetes in 30 days by living a raw food lifestyle. *www.foodmatters.tv/_webapp/Movie_Store.*

References and Book Resource List

❋ *Breaking the Food Seduction: The Hidden Reasons Behind Food Cravings and 7 Steps to End Them Naturally* by Neal Barnard, MD.

❋ *Diet for a New America: How Your Food Choices Affect Your Health, Happiness and the Future of Life on Earth* by John Robbins.

❋ *Disease-Proof Your Child: Feeding Kids Right* by Joel Fuhrman, MD.

❋ *Eat, Drink and Be Vegan* by Dreena Burton.

❋ *Eat to Live* by Joel Fuhrman, MD and Mehmet Oz, MD.

❋ *Excitotoxins: The Taste That Kills* by Russell L. Blaylock, MD.

❋ *Fast Food Nation: The Dark Side of the All-American Meal* by Eric Schlosser.

❋ *Fats That Heal Fats That Kill* by Udo Erasmus.

❋ *Feeding the Whole Family: Whole Foods Recipes for Babies, Young Children and Their Parents* by Cynthia Lair.

❋ *Food, Inc.* edited by Karl Weber *www.takepart.com/foodinc*

❋ *Food Allergy Survival Guide* by Vesanto Melina, MS, RD, Jo Stepaniak, MSEd, and Dina Aronson, MS, RD.

❋ *Food Politics: How the Food Industry Influences Nutrition and Health* by Marion Nestle.

❋ *Genetic Nutritioneering* by Jeffrey Bland, Ph.D.

❋ *Get the Sugar Out: 501 Simple Ways to Cut the Sugar Out of Any Diet* by Ann Louise Gittleman, MS, CNS.

❋ *Green For Life* by Victoria Boutenko.

❋ *Heaven on Earth: A Handbook for Parents of Young Children* by Sharifa Oppenheimer. (As referenced with the *Cinnamon Spice Birthday Cake* on page 152.) *www.ourheavenonearth.net.*

❋ *How It All Vegan!* by Sarah Kramer and Tanya Barnard.

❋ *In Defense of Food: An Eater's Manifesto* by Michael Pollan.

❋ *Nourishing Traditions* by Sally Fallon and Mary Enig.

❋ *Nourishing Wisdom: A Mind-Body Approach to Nutrition and Well-Being* by Marc David.

❋ *Superfoods* by David Wolfe.

❋ *Sweet Deception* by Dr. Joseph Mercola.

❋ *The China Study* by T. Colin Campbell, Ph.D. & Thomas M. Campbell II.

❋ *The Feel Good Food Guide* by Deborah Page Johnson.

❋ *The Food Revolution: How Your Diet Can Help Save Your Life and the World* by John Robbins.

❋ *The Metabolic Typing Diet* by William Wolcott, et.al.

❋ *The Real Food Daily Cookbook* by Ann Gentry.

❋ *The Stevia Cookbook* by Ray Sahelian, MD and Donna Gates.

❋ *The Stevia Story: A Tale of Incredible Sweetness & Intrigue* by Bill and Linda Bonvie and Donna Gates.

❋ *There is a Cure for Diabetes* by Gabriel Cousens, MD.

❋ *The UltraMind Solution: The Simple Way to Defeat Depression, Overcome Anxiety and Sharpen Your Mind* by Mark Hyman, MD.

Please see www.vigdorhess.com and *www.SweetnessWithoutSugar.com* for more suggested resources.

Additional Websites and Reading Resources

❋ Physicians Committee for Responsible Medicine (PCRM): *www.pcrm.org* or 202.686.2210.

❋ Center for Science in the Public Interest (CSPI) Nutrition Action Healthletter: *www.cspinet.org* or 202.332.9110.

❋ Vegetarian Times: *www.vegetariantimes.com*.

❋ Nancy Appleton, Ph.D. offers information about the negative effects of sugar consumption: *www.NancyAppleton.com*.

Bibliography

❋ Adams, M. Campaign for commercial-free childhood blasts TV promotion of junk foods to children. *http://www.newstarget.com/021835.html*.

❋ Alvarez, et al. Effect of aqueous extract of stevia rebaudiana bertone on biochemical parameters of normal adult persons. *Brazilian J Med Biol Res*, 1986, 19:771-774.

❋ Ballew, C. et al. Beverage choices affect adequacy of children's nutrient intakes. *Archives of Pediatric and Adolescent Medicine* 2000, 154: 1148-1152.

❋ Bantle JP, Raatz SK, Thomas W, Georgopoulos A. Effects of dietary fructose on plasma lipids in healthy subjects. *Am. J. Clin. Nutr, 2000, 72 (5): 1128–34. PMID 11063439.*

❋ Campbell TC, Caedo JP, Jr., Bulatao-Jayme J, et al. Aflatoxin M in human urine. *Nature*, 1970, 227: 403-404.

❋ Centers for Disease Control and Prevention. National diabetes fact sheet: general information and national estimates on diabetes in the united states, 2000. Atlanta, GA: Centers for Disease Control and Prevention.

❋ Colditz, GA. Economic costs of obesity and inactivity. *Med. Sci. Sports Exerc.*, 1999, 31: S663-S667.

❋ Coulstron, A.M. The role of dietary fats in plant-based diets. *Am J Clin Nutr,* 1999, 70 (Supp):512S-15S.

❋ Dennison BA, Rockwell HL, Baker SL. Excess fruit juice consumption by preschool-aged children is associated with short stature and obesity. *Pediatrics, 1997, 99 (1): 15–22. PMID 8989331.*

❋ Dhingra R, Sullivan L, Jacques PF, et al. Soft drink consumption and risk of developing cardiometabolic risk factors and the metabolic syndrome in middle-aged adults in the community. *Circulation,* 2007, 116:480-488.

❀ Dietz, WH. Health consequences of obesity in youth: childhood predictors of adult disease. *Pediatrics*, 1998, 101: 518-525.

❀ Drewnowski A., Krahn DD, Demitrack MA, Nairn K, Gosnell BA. Taste responses and preferences for sweet high-fat foods: evidence for opioid involvement. *Physiol Behav*, 1992, 51:371-9.

❀ Elliott SS, Keim NL, Stern JS, Teff K, Havel PJ. Fructose, weight gain, and the insulin resistance syndrome. *Am. J. Clin. Nutr., November 2002*, 76 (5): 911–22. PMID 12399260. *http://www.ajcn.org/cgi/content/full/76/5/911.*

❀ Flegal KM, Carroll MD, Ogden CI., et al. Prevalence and trends in obesity among U.S. adults, 1999-2000. *JAMA*, 2002, 288: 1723-1727.

❀ Fontaine KR, and Barofsky I. Obesity and health-related quality of life. *Obesity Rev.*, 2001, 2: 173-182.

❀ Hamann, A. and Matthaei, S. Regulation of energy balance by leptin. *Exp Clin Endocrinol Diabetes*, 1996, 104:293-300.

❀ Harnack, L. et al. Soft drink consumption among US children and adolescents: nutritional consequences. *Journal of the American Dietetic Association*, 1999, 99: 436-441.

❀ International Diabetes Federation. Diabetes epidemic out of control. December 4, 2006. *http://www.idf.org/home/index.cfm?node=1563.*

❀ Isganaitis E, Lustig RH. Fast food, central nervous system insulin resistance, and obesity. *Arterioscler. Thromb. Vasc. Biol.*, 2005, 25 (12): 2451–62. *doi:10.1161/01. ATV.0000186208.06964.91. PMID 16166564.*

❀ Jacobson, M. Liquid candy: how soft drinks are harming Americans' health. *Center for Science in the Public Interest*, 1998, Washington, DC.

❀ Ji, Sayer. The dark side of wheat: new perspectives on celiac disease and wheat intolerance. *http://www.greenmedinfo.com/ page/dark-side-wheat-new-perspectives-celiac-disease-wheat-intolerance-sayer-ji.*

✳ Ji, Sayer. Opening pandora's bread box: the critical role of wheat lectin in human disease. *http://www.greenmedinfo.com/content/opening-pandoras-bread-box-critical-role-wheat-lectin-human-disease.*

✳ Johnson RK, Appel LJ, Brands M, et al. Dietary sugars intake and cardiovascular health: a scientific statement from the American Heart Association. *Circulation*, 2009, 120:1011-1020.

✳ Kostraba JN, Cruickshanks KJ, Lawler-Heavner J, et al. Early exposure to cow's milk and solid foods in infancy, genetic predisposition, and risk of IDDM. *Diabetes*, 1993, 42: 288-295.

✳ Lardinois, C.K. The role of omega-3 fatty acids on insulin secretion and insulin sensitivity. *Med Hypotheses*, 1997, 24(3): 243-48.

✳ Ludwig DS, Pereira MA, Kroenke CH, et al. Dietary fiber, weight gain, and cardiovascular disease risk factors in young adults. *JAMA*, 1999, 282:1539-46.

✳ Ludwig, DS, Peterson, KE, and Gorthaker, SI. Relation between consumption of sugar-sweetened drinks and childhood obesity: a prospective, observational analysis. *The Lancet*, 2001, 357: 505-508.

✳ Lustig, Robert H., MD. Childhood obesity: behavioral aberration or biochemical drive? Reinterpreting the first law of thermodynamics. *Nature Clinical Practice, Endocrinology & Metabolism Review*, August 2006, 2;8:447-457.

✳ Lustig, Robert H., MD. The 'skinny' on childhood obesity: how our western environment starves kids' brains. *Pediatric Annals*, November 2006, 35;12:899-907.

✳ Madhavan TV, and Gopalan C. The effect of dietary protein on carcinogenesis of aflatoxin. *Arch. Path.*, 1968, 85: 133-137.

✳ McManamy, J. Depression and diabetes. *http://www.mcmanweb.com/article-42.htm.*

✳ National Research Council, National Academy of Sciences. Pesticides in the diets of infants and children. *National Academy Press*, 1993, 184-185. Washington, DC.

✳ Ogden, CI., Fegal KM, Carroll MD, et al. Prevalence and trends in overweight among U.S. children and adolescents. *JAMA*, 2002, 288: 1728-1732.

✳ Seyfried, Thomas N., Shelton, Laura M. Cancer as a metabolic disease. *Nutrition and Metabolism*, 2010, 7:7. *http://www. nutritionandmetabolism.com/content/7/1/7*.

✳ Simopoulos, A.P. Essential fatty acids in health and chronic disease. *Am J Clin Nutr.*, 1990, 70 (Supp):560S-69S.

✳ Stiles, Steve. Added sugars in diet linked to higher triglycerides, lower HDL-C in NHANES data. *Medscape Today*. April 2010. *http://www.medscape.com/viewarticle/720588?sssdmh=dm1.613 092&src=nldne&uac=66422BV*.

✳ Teff, KL; Elliott SS, Tschöp M, Kieffer TJ, Rader D, Heiman M, Townsend RR, Keim NL, D'Alessio D, Havel PJ. Dietary fructose reduces circulating insulin and leptin, attenuates postprandial suppression of ghrelin, and increases triglycerides in women. *J Clin Endocrinol Metab.*, June 2004, 89 (6): 2963–72. *doi:10.1210/jc.2003-031855. PMID 15181085.*

✳ Tuomisto T, Hetheringon MM, Morris MF, Tuomisto MT, Turjanmaa V, Lapalainen R. Psychological and physiological characteristics of sweet food "addiction." *Int J Eat Disord.*, 1999, 25:169-75.

✳ Wang, G., and Dietz, W. Economic burden of obesity in youths aged 6 to 17 years: 1979-1999. *Pediatrics*, 2002, 109: e81.

✳ Welsh, JA, Sharma, A, Abramson JL, et.al. Caloric sweetener consumption and dyslipidemia among US adults. *JAMA*, 2010, 303(15):1490-1497. *http://jama.ama-assn.org/cgi/content/ short/303/15/1490*.

✳ World Diabetes Foundation. "Diabetes facts." *http://www. worlddiabetesfoundation.org/composite-35.htm*.

✳ Wylie-Rosett, Judith; et al. Carbohydrates and increases in obesity: does the type of carbohydrate make a difference? *Obesity Res*, 2004, 12: 124S–129S. *doi:10.1038/oby.2004.277. http:// www.obesityresearch.org/cgi/content/full/12/suppl_2/124S*.

About

the Author

Wendy Vigdor-Hess earned a Bachelor of Science degree from Indiana University and completed traditional training in nutrition at Loyola University. She attained her dietetic internship through Bastyr University. Nationally certified as a registered dietitian, Wendy also became a certified WellCoach®. A staunch believer in the importance of exercise and its relationship to wellness, Wendy has been certified by the American Council on Exercise since 1994.

In addition to her private practice, Wendy has worked as a public health nutritionist for the Women, Infants and Children Program (WIC) in Seattle, Washington before settling in Virginia in 2003. She has consulted with The ARC (Association of Retarded Citizens) of the Piedmont (in Virginia) as well as with The Johns Hopkins Integrative Medicine and Digestive Center (in Maryland). On a regular basis, Wendy also speaks to local and national audiences about a range of nutrition and wellness topics.

For nearly 20 years, Wendy has practiced in the health field as a registered dietitian, integrative nutritional counselor, WellCoach® and Reiki master teacher. She uses an individualized approach that allows her to address and specialize in a variety of health issues.

Wendy encourages her clients and students to "dream big" to reach the goals they most desire and to connect with their innate, empowered selves. Through counseling, writing and teaching, she shares this knowledge and passion for healthy and vibrant living.

With husband, Bill, son, Solomon, daughter, Althea, and dog, Maude, Wendy enjoys hiking, yoga, creating, dancing and get-togethers with friends. Experience has shown her how dramatically nutrition, energy healing and movement can improve the quality of life for individuals, children and families.

Acknowledgements

My heartfelt, eternal gratitude and love to my husband, Bill, for your generous heart, patience, kindness, compassion, support, gentle nudges, shared parenting and willingness to taste the "mistakes" and experiments along the way. For seeing my potential many years ago and standing beside me. Our journey has led us and our family to new places of sweetness. Thank you for sharing it all with me and keeping me laughing.

Deepest thanks to many of you who knew I would write before I did. Included in this list are Dini Mari, Karen Raden and Stephen and Laura Bruno. Not only did you believe I would write, you believed in me. Enormous thanks to all of you for your encouragement, love and support through the years.

Special thanks to Traci Moore (*www.tracimoore.org*) for midwifing me through this process! Your amazing editorial expertise, patience, suggestions and support have been appreciated beyond measure. Your innate sweetness shines through each word.

Enormous thanks to Gwen Gades (*www.beapurplepenguin.com*) for your sense of humor, playfulness and talent in designing the interior of this book.

Immense gratitude to Jasper Burns (*www.jasperburns.com*) for his willingness to participate in this project in its mid-designed state. Your expertise, efficiency, patience, sense of calm, generosity and love are a fitting end to the birth of this book.

Sweet thanks to Sherry Sraddha Van Dyke (*http://sraddha.weebly.com/*) for the beautiful photos of my recipes, for your faith and enthusiasm in this delicious process and for the gift of gratitude in manifesting what is in our hearts. Thank you also to my in-laws, Betsy and George Hess, and to our neighbors, Linda and Ann, for loaning some of the dishware used in these photos.

Gratitude to Jan Gulley Gerdin (*www.bring-design.com*) for taking my vision for SolThea Press and giving it organic form while adding your own creative flair, heart, metaphoric design and expertise.

Many thanks to Mom and Dad, Louise and Justin. You gave me fond memories of sweetness. I embraced Mom's love of chocolate and decadent desserts, and Dad's preference for fruit. I remember sharing with Dad the apples he cut in the apple slicer, and singing in the kitchen with Mom as we made chocolate mousse. In many ways, you supported and informed my journey toward sweetness.

Thanks to Laura Bruno for your friendship, editing and coaching advice, compassion, inspiration, faith and our continued "mutual blessings". Many years ago, a wise man alluded to the blessings to be shared between us. I am grateful beyond words that he was right and that both of you are in my life.

Thank you to Sarah Kramer and Tanya Barnard for giving me permission to include variations of your recipes and make them gluten-free. Many blessings to you for sharing your delicious vittles and great books.

An offering of thanks to Pat Leavitt, for your wonderful suggestions, contributions and testings. For your nourishment and love......

Continued gratitude to Maia Oden (*www.cdbaby.com/Artist/MaiaOden*), for sharing your melodies, beautiful songs, love of nature, sense of innocence and Goddess strength. For sharing all of this and more with our family. We are blessed.

Many thanks to Katherine Gray for your enthusiasm, positive attitude, recipe testing and genuine care and love for our children.

Thank you to Marley Peale for your generosity, time and efficiency. I'm grateful for your help analyzing the nutrient content for many of the recipes. I look forward to working with you in the nutritional field.

I'd like to acknowledge all of you who have been a part of my *Sweetness Without Sugar* classes, offered feedback on my desserts or recipes, or contributed ideas for some of your favorite recipes. Thank you for your patience during the completion of this second edition.

And finally, my love to Solomon and Althea, our children, for your constant reflection, insight, unconditional love, patience and trust. Thank you for choosing me as your Mother. May we always find fun and sweetness in our lives— both together and as you embark on your own paths. (We'll be cheering for you!) You inspire me every day.

LIST OF RECIPES

The recipes in this section are raw versions of recipes included above *and* they are recipes that can be enjoyed while also following a raw food lifestyle.

RAW AND SUPERFOOD TREATS (continued)

LIST OF ALLERGEN-FREE RECIPES

CORN-FREE RECIPES

All of the recipes are corn-free though some (as indicated in the actual recipes) include ingredients that may be corn-derived.

NUT- OR SEED-FREE RECIPES

Some of the recipes in this list include nuts. If desired, seeds or seed butters may be substituted for nuts.

NUT- OR SEED-FREE RECIPES (continued)

NUT- OR SEED-FREE RAW RECIPES

NUT- AND SEED-FREE RECIPES

Flax seed and chia seeds are used in some of the recipes on this list.

NUT- AND SEED-FREE RECIPES (continued)

NUT- AND SEED-FREE RAW RECIPES

SOY-FREE RECIPES

SOY-FREE RECIPES (continued)

SOY-FREE RAW RECIPES

INDEX